FEAR
LESS

To my darling Bunny.

Lyla, you are my inspiration.

The day you came into my life,
I was given purpose, direction
and unconditional love.

FEAR
LESS

TRINNY WOODALL

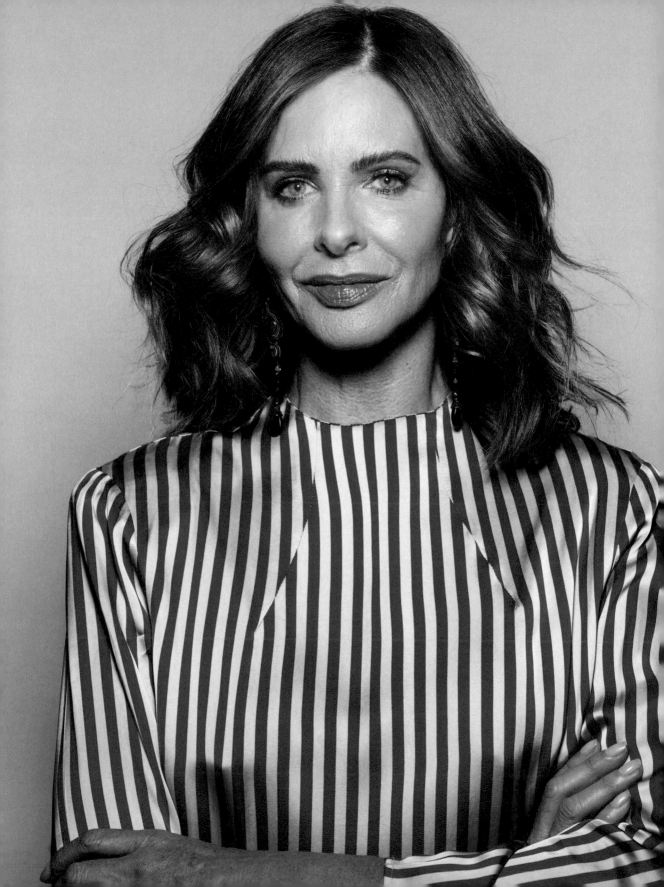

Contents

TAKE A
LEAP OF

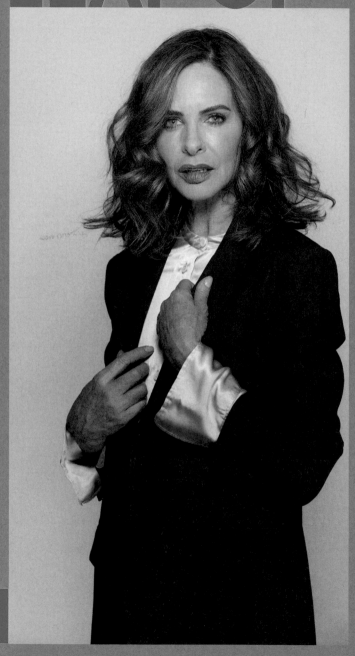

FAITH

What this book will do for you

In *FEARLESS* I am going to show you what life has taught me on my journey to becoming fearless.

I will be covering life, beauty and style so that you can take a truly holistic approach. Some of this will resonate with you and some won't, though all have mattered to me. We are all starting from different places and are held back by different things in our lives. I want to get you to the stage where you fearlessly project energy into the world, and you feel the world respond.

I have spent much of my career trying to help women feel good about themselves. Putting on clothes that make you feel great, caring for your skin and wearing makeup that enhances your natural beauty are not frivolous extras – they are outward projections of energy and confidence. We will also look at the elements that will make you feel more confident on the inside, the things that will allow you to have faith in yourself and your choices.

When the woman you see in the mirror looks energised and confident, it gives you the momentum to stride purposefully through your day without fear. Let's begin.

Push forward and do it anyway

FEAR
LESS

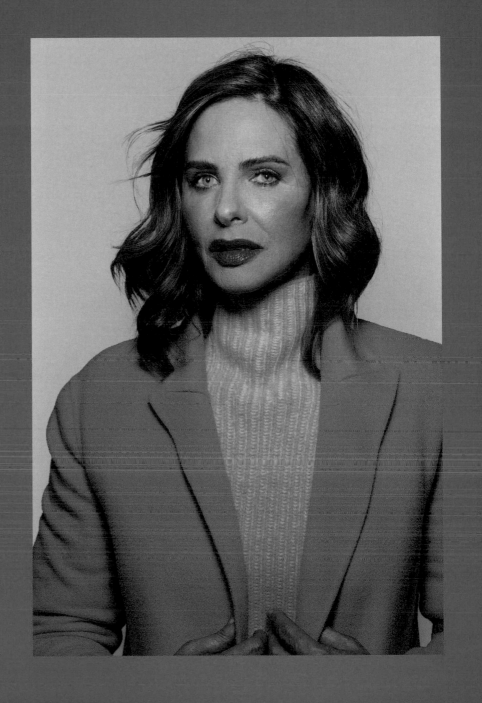

IDENTIFY

UNDERSTAND THE COLOURS

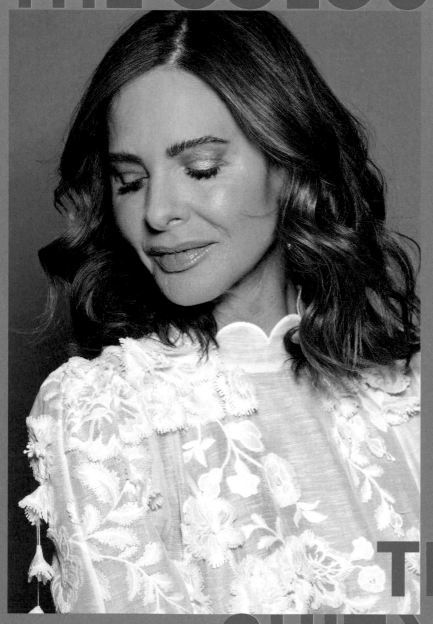

THAT SUIT YOU

How to work out what will suit you

In this section, we will be using multiple tools to find out what suits you best. These aren't hard and fast rules, rather a guide to help you in your decisions and to see what really suits you.

What I have learnt over the years is that if we can correctly identify our colouring and skin type, we will be able to shop for clothing, makeup and skincare with far more ease. Knowing what suits you removes a big barrier and allows you to build confidence in how you dress and present yourself.

How many of us have been in a shop and fallen in love with the shape of a piece of clothing and then hesitated over the colour? If you already know what colours suit you, you would either rush to buy it or easily cast it aside, you wouldn't need to waste time debating. The same applies to skincare. Many people buy skincare according to their mood, the smell of a product or the joy of a texture. But if you truly know your skin type, and you understand the skin issues you might want to be addressing, focusing in on the products that will really transform your skin will save you money. And I don't think I know one woman who only owns the makeup she uses. Stop being drawn in by a new colour of lipstick or blush, and instead pick the colours that will suit you.

When you know how to look after your skin as well as the right combination of makeup for you, and you couple this with the knowledge of the clothing colours that suit you, you give yourself the tools to put yourself together with complete ease and confidence. Every woman deserves to be able to leave their fear behind on what does and does not suit them.

Knowing what suits you removes a big barrier

Your skin type

It can be tricky to identify your skin type, but it is absolutely worth taking the time to do so. It will ensure that all the skincare tweaks you make will actually work for you, as you will be able to select the right products for your skin type and your concerns (see page 124). Below are the bookends of your skincare routine according to your skin type. Embrace the skin you are in.

Dry

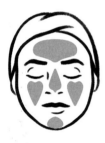

Your skin will feel tight and dry all over. The skin will have no surface oiliness and it might have extra dryness on the cheeks. If you throw water on your face, your skin will feel tight as it dries. The essential products for you to use are:

- Cleansing balm
- PHA or AHA exfoliating liquid
- Nourishing moisturiser

Oily

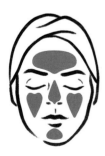

Your skin will feel oily, especially the T-zone, and you will have visible pores. There will be an all over sense of oiliness by the middle of your day, with your skin and especially your forehead looking oily. The essential products for you to use are:

- Cleansing gel or wash
- BHA or AHA exfoliating liquid
- Oil balancing moisturiser

Normal

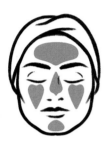

Your skin will feel comfortable; not too oily or too dry. You will have no surface oil on your face and no really dry patches. When you put water on your face and let it dry, it will feel fine. The essential products for you to use are:

- Cleansing balm or gel
- PHA or AHA exfoliating liquid
- Light moisturiser

Combination

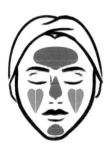

Your skin will feel oily in your T-zone and drier on your cheeks. Combination is exactly what it says on the tin. There will be oiliness especially on the forehead, around your nose and around your mouth. You might have visible pores and your cheeks might be normal or a bit dry. The essential products for you to use are:

- Cleansing balm or gel
- BHA or AHA exfoliating liquid

Now you know your skin type, you can go to the **BEAUTY** section (see page 102) and decide your main skin concerns. You can then select the right products for the skin you have today. There is nothing to be afraid of when you know your skin and can achieve the right routine for you.

Your **cleanser** and **moisturiser** should be based on **your skin type**. Your **serum** should be based on **your skin concern**. Your **acid** should be based on either your **skin type or your concern**.

What shape is your face?

It is useful to determine your face shape, to help pick glasses, jewellery and hats, and work out how best to apply your makeup.

Look at a photo of your face taken front on with your hair pulled back or off your face. Using a coloured pen (so it stands out), draw around your face. You can do this on your smartphone too. From this outline you can determine what your face shape is. It is also worth thinking about if you have a long or short forehead in relation to the rest of your face.

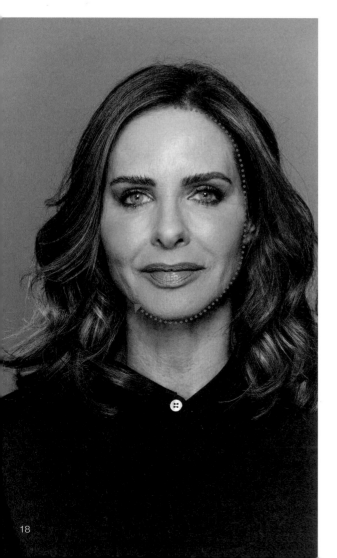

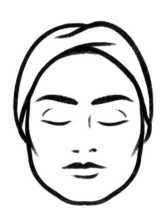

Square

Square faces feature a forehead, cheekbones and jawline that are the same width. You will probably also have a well-defined jawline.

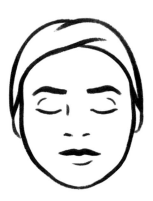

Round

Round faces have wide foreheads, full cheeks and a round chin.

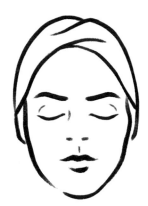

Oval

Oval faces are longer than they are wide and they tend to have well-proportioned features.

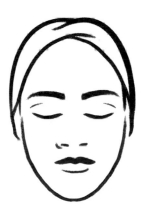

Long Oval

A long oval face is longer than it is wide. Typically, your forehead will be the widest past of your face and your features will be soft. You might have narrower eyes.

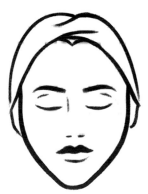

Heart

Heart-shaped faces have a wider forehead and more pronounced chin. Your hairline will be V-shaped or you have a widow's peak, though the features of your face are rounded.

Defining your colours: skin, hair and eyes

You should base the answers on your skin, eye and current hair colour (the colour that frames your face). There will always be variations, so select those that you feel represent you best. You will then use the numbers on these pages as a tool to identify your dominant overall tone. For even more detail, go to **trinnylondon.com**

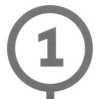

SKIN TONE

Ignore the hair, eye, ethnicity, gender and age in the following images to find your closest skin tone match. We have split them into seven categories, and within those there are options to identify yourself. Consider that our skin is made up of a multitude of colours and our undertones can contain warm colours (reds, oranges, yellows) and cool colours (blues, greens and purples).

Lightest

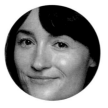 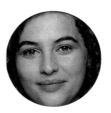 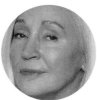

Alabaster	Porcelain	Peaches + cream light	Pale pink tones
I have a cool/neutral undertone, I burn easily.	I have a neutral undertone. I can go in the sun a little without burning.	I have neutral /peachy undertones. My skin is quite consistent all year round.	I have slightly pink undertones and may have sensitive skin. I burn easily.
2 points	**3 points**	**3 points**	**4 points**

Light

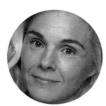

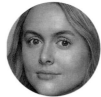

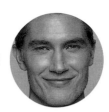

Porcelain olive

I have neutral/olive undertones. I have the ability to burn, but I also can tan.

3 points

Peaches + cream

I have neutral undertones and my skin is quite consistent all year.

3 points

Pale olive

I have cool /neutral olive undertones. I may have a few freckles. I can tan.

2 points

Light Medium

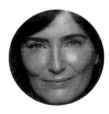

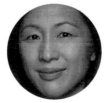

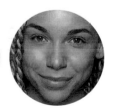

Rosy olive

I have neutral/rosy undertones. My skin always has a rosy flush and I can tan.

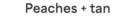

3 points

Peaches + tan

I have neutral undertones. I will burn if I don't wear SPF.

3 points

Olive

I have neutral olive undertones. My skin can feel dull in the winter.

2 points

Light tan

I have neutral/golden undertones. I tan deeply and don't burn easily.

3 points

Honey

I have golden undertones all year round. I can tan without burning.

2 points

Medium

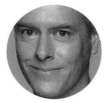 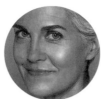 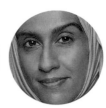 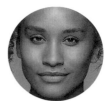

Rosy red	**Dark tan**	**Dark olive**	**Deep honey**
I have rosy undertones and can burn easily. I have a consistent flush.	I have tan/ golden undertones all year round and can easily tan.	I have neutral/olive undertones. My skin can look dull in winter, but I tan easily.	I have golden undertones all year round. I tan without burning.
2 points	**2** points	**2** points	**3** points

Medium Deep

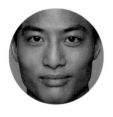 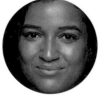 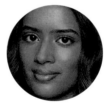 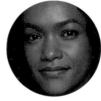 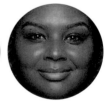

Caramel	**Golden caramel**	**Dark caramel**	**Toffee**	**Deep caramel**
I have neutral undertones. My skin can feel dull in winter, but tan easily in the sun.	I have golden undertones. My skin is consistent and I tan fairly easily.	I have cool/neutral undertones. I can have an uneven tone around my eyes. I tan easily.	I have neutral undertones. When I tan, my skin can look bronzed for a long time.	I have neutral/golden undertones. My skin is even and I tan easily.
3 points	**2** points	**2** points	**3** points	**2** points

Deep

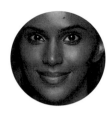 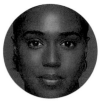 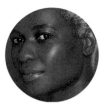 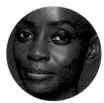

Deepest caramel

I have neutral/golden undertones. My skin changes throughout the year.

3 points

Deep toffee

I have neutral/warm undertones. My skin can have dark circles, but is consistent.

4 points

Nutmeg

I have yellow undertones. I can look very bronzed when I tan.

3 points

Chestnut

I have neutral/warm undertones. My skin is consistent all year round.

3 points

Deepest

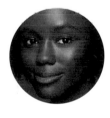 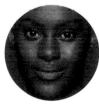 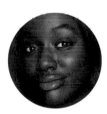 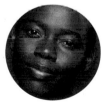

Deep chestnut

I have slightly red undertones and I can burn fairly easily.

4 points

Deep cinnamon

I have neutral undertones and my skin is consistent all year round.

3 points

Ebony

I have neutral undertones. I tan quickly and have an even complexion.

3 points

Deep ebony

I have cool/neutral undertones. My skin is even, but it can look dull in the winter.

2 points

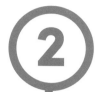

HAIR COLOUR

You should only consider your current hair colour here. You want to match your colour to the hair that currently frames your face, even if dyed. If you have grey hair it won't be flat grey, so use the colour that is closest to your current tone of grey.

Brunette/Black

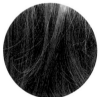
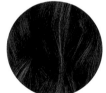
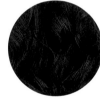

Mousy	Tawny	Warm brunette	Brunette	Dark brown
3 points	**4** points	**4** points	**3** points	**3** points

Darkest brown	Black
2 points	**1** points

Redhead

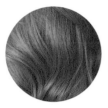 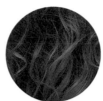 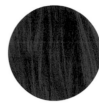 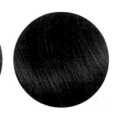

Strawberry blonde

Auburn

Copper blonde

Red

Deep red

4 points

5 points

4 points

5 points

5 points

Bronde

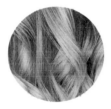 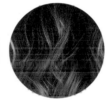

Cool bronde

Neutral bronde

Warm bronde

2 points

3 points

4 points

Blonde

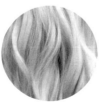 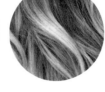 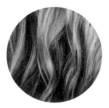

Cool blonde

Dirty cool blonde

Warm blonde

2 points

3 points

4 points

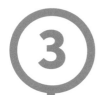

EYE COLOUR

Now look solely at your eye colour. Don't factor in eye shape or skin tone. You will either need to look in a mirror in good light to see this clearly, or even better - ask a friend to help!

Blue

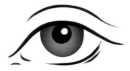

Your eye is bright blue, with a deeper, darker blue around the outside.

 point

Your eye is clear blue, with no variation in colour.

 points

Your eye is a dirty blue, with elements of grey.

 points

Green

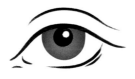

Your eye is bright green, with a deeper, darker green around the outside.

 point

Your eye is a clear green, with no variation in colour.

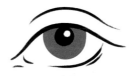 **points**

Your eye is a dirty green, with elements of other colours, but not hazel.

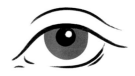 **points**

Brown

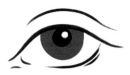 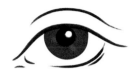 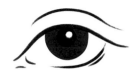

Your eye is a cool, light solid brown.

3 points

Your eye has flecks of warm orange in the brown.

4 points

Your eye is a very dark, single shade of brown.

3 points

Grey

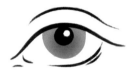 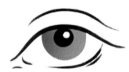 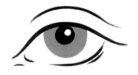

Grey with elements of blue.

3 points

Grey, with elements of green.

3 points

Your eye is a solid grey.

1 point

Hazel

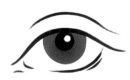 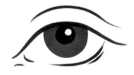

A combination of green and brown - a majority of green.

3 points

A combination of green and brown - a majority of brown.

4 points

Your results

Now that you have selected your closest matches for your skin, hair and eye, you should have three unique numbers. I want you to add these numbers together to get your total. For example, I am:

1. SKIN TONE	= Light Medium, Rosy Olive	= 3 points
2. HAIR COLOUR	= Brunette, Tawny	= 4 points
3. EYE COLOUR	= Clear Blue	= 2 points
TOTAL	= **NEUTRAL**	= **9 points**

Now look at the table below and right to find your total score and discover your natural tone. There are 5 categories here and you will naturally sit in one more than any other.

Knowing whether we are Cool, Cool/neutral, Neutral, Warm/neutral or Warm will influence all of our colour decisions going forward. Throughout the book I have also flagged the options that will suit each tone best, so that you can always feel fearless in your choices and learn how to curate your own palettes.

Who you are

Cool

If your skin has more blues, greens and purples in it, then it is cool. Your hair might be black or cool blonde and your eyes will likely be bright blue or green or a solid grey. You will suit silver jewellery.

Cool/neutral

If your skin tone has some blue in it and you generally don't tan well, you will have cool/neutral tones. You will have a low level of contrast, so your hair might be cool in shade and your eyes will be bright and clear. You will suit silver but can wear gold jewellery.

Neutral

If your skin has an equal balance of the shades and it is quite consistent all year round, then your tone is neutral. Your hair will have warmer tones to it and your eyes will likely have depth and variation in colour. You will suit both silver and gold jewellery.

 Warm/neutral

If your skin tone has a little bit of warmth in it, in the form of pink or rosy, then it is warm/neutral. Your eyes will likely be dirty or dark and your hair might be warm in tone and darker. You will suit gold jewellery, but can wear silver.

Warm

If you have more reds, oranges and yellows and no coolness to your skin, then it is warm. You will have a lot of warmth and redness in your hair and your eyes will be very dark, hazel or brown with warm flecks. You will suit gold jewellery.

Cool palette

Now you know you are cool in tone, here is a quick reference guide to some of your best shades. Use this as a guide to curate the colours you wear and as inspiration for how you can pair and contrast them too.

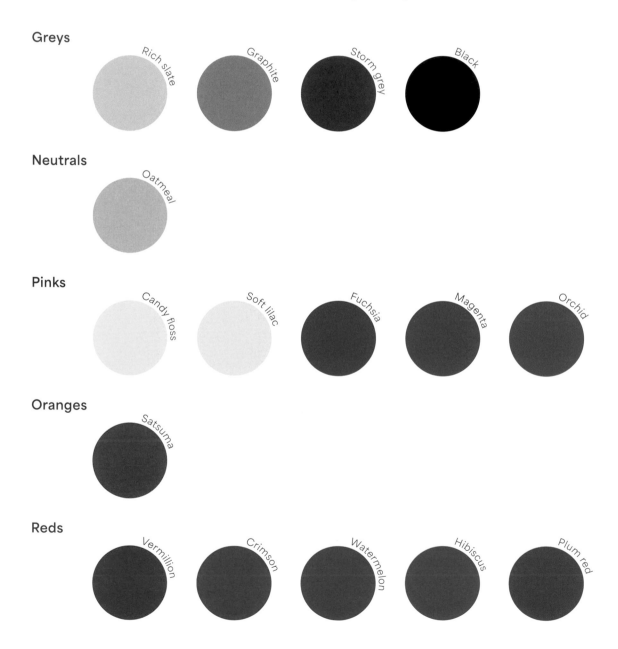

Greys

Rich slate Graphite Storm grey Black

Neutrals

Oatmeal

Pinks

Candy floss Soft lilac Fuchsia Magenta Orchid

Oranges

Satsuma

Reds

Vermillion Crimson Watermelon Hibiscus Plum red

Purples

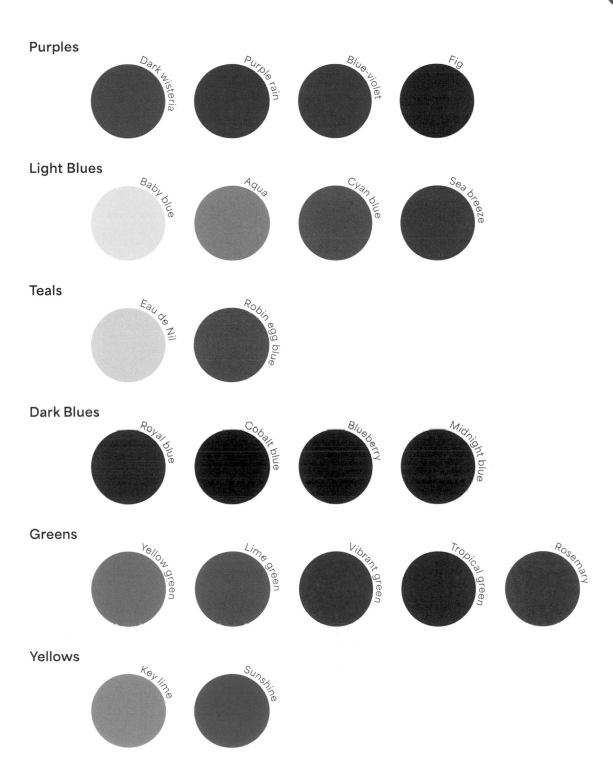

Dark wisteria   Purple rain   Blue-violet   Fig

Light Blues

Baby blue   Aqua   Cyan blue   Sea breeze

Teals

Eau de Nil   Robin egg blue

Dark Blues

Royal blue   Cobalt blue   Blueberry   Midnight blue

Greens

Yellow green   Lime green   Vibrant green   Tropical green   Rosemary

Yellows

Key lime   Sunshine

Cool/neutral palette

Now you know you are cool/neutral in tone, here is a quick reference guide to some of your best shades. Use this as a guide to curate the colours you wear and as inspiration for how you can pair and contrast them too.

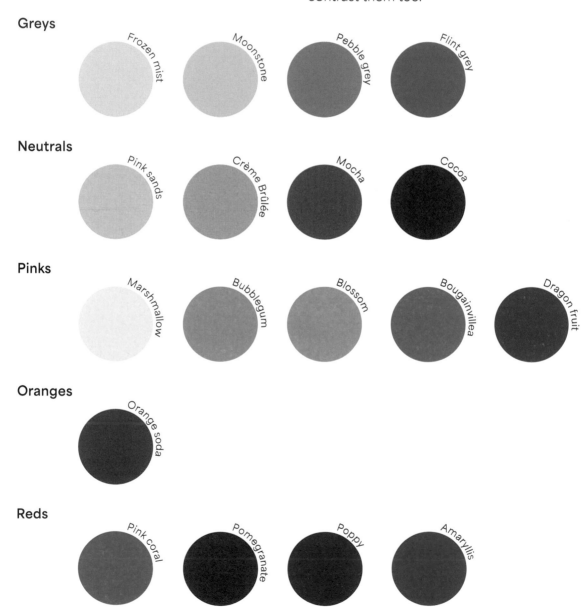

Greys

Frozen mist · Moonstone · Pebble grey · Flint grey

Neutrals

Pink sands · Crème Brûlée · Mocha · Cocoa

Pinks

Marshmallow · Bubblegum · Blossom · Bougainvillea · Dragon fruit

Oranges

Orange soda

Reds

Pink coral · Pomegranate · Poppy · Amaryllis

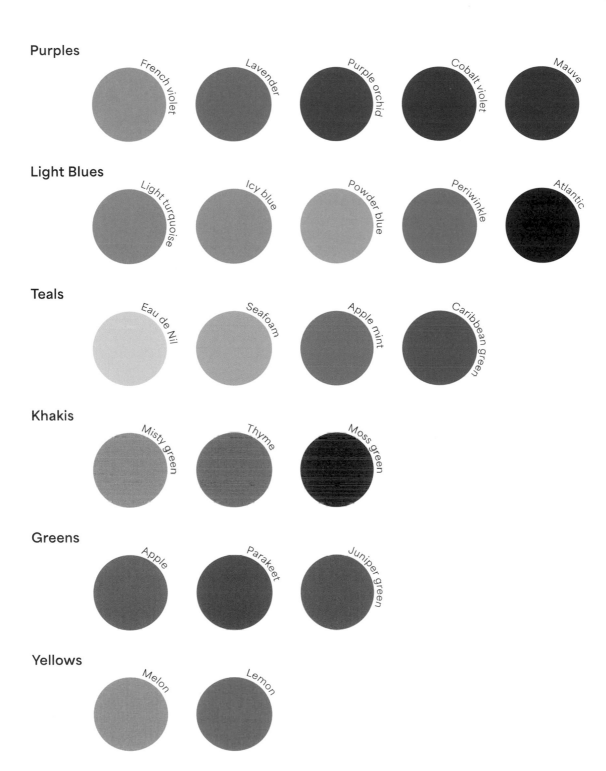

Purples

French violet

Lavender

Purple orchid

Cobalt violet

Mauve

Light Blues

Light turquoise

Icy blue

Powder blue

Periwinkle

Atlantic

Teals

Eau de Nil

Seafoam

Apple mint

Caribbean green

Khakis

Misty green

Thyme

Moss green

Greens

Apple

Parakeet

Juniper green

Yellows

Melon

Lemon

Neutral palette

Now you know you are neutral in tone, here is a quick reference guide to some of your best shades. Use this as a guide to curate the colours you wear and as inspiration for how you can pair and contrast them too.

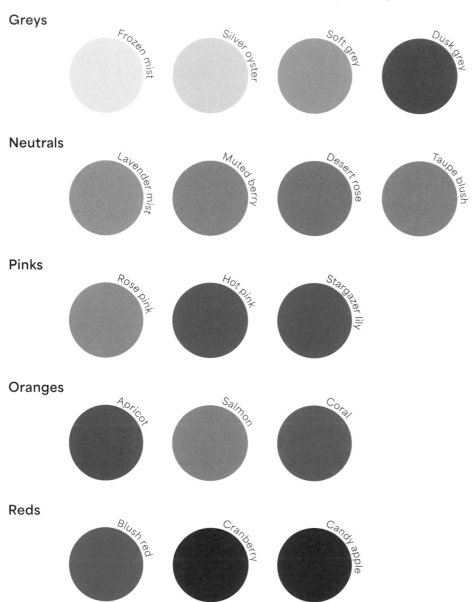

Greys

Frozen mist | Silver oyster | Soft grey | Dusk grey

Neutrals

Lavender mist | Muted berry | Desert rose | Taupe blush

Pinks

Rose pink | Hot pink | Stargazer lily

Oranges

Apricot | Salmon | Coral

Reds

Blush red | Cranberry | Candy apple

Purples

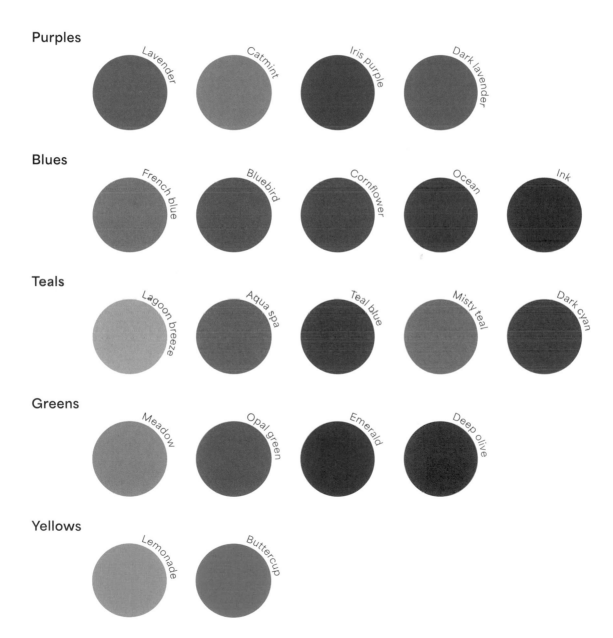

Lavender

Catmint

Iris purple

Dark lavender

Blues

French blue

Bluebird

Cornflower

Ocean

Ink

Teals

Lagoon breeze

Aqua spa

Teal blue

Misty teal

Dark cyan

Greens

Meadow

Opal green

Emerald

Deep olive

Yellows

Lemonade

Buttercup

Warm/neutral palette

Now you know you are warm/neutral in tone, here is a quick reference guide to some of your best shades. Use this as a guide to curate the colours you wear and as inspiration for how you can pair and contrast them too.

Greys

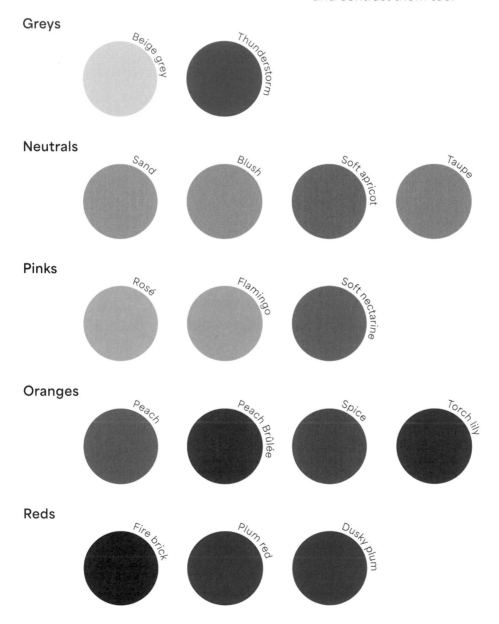

Beige grey

Thunderstorm

Neutrals

Sand

Blush

Soft apricot

Taupe

Pinks

Rosé

Flamingo

Soft nectarine

Oranges

Peach

Peach Brûlée

Spice

Torch lily

Reds

Fire brick

Plum red

Dusky plum

Purples

Amethyst   Purple rain   Aubergine

Light Blues

Nordic sky   Royal navy   Deep cobalt   Deep teal

Teals

Aquamarine   Aqua pearl   Robin egg blue   Sea green

Khakis

Khaki

Greens

Spearmint   Pine green   Velvet teal   Forest

Yellows

Pineapple   Amber   Daffodil

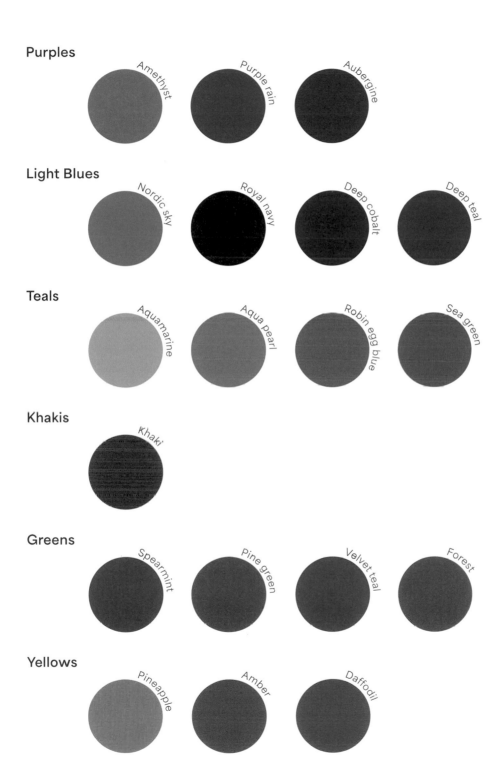

Warm palette

Now you know you are warm in tone, here is a quick reference guide to some of your best shades. Use this as a guide to curate the colours you wear and as inspiration for how you can pair and contrast them too.

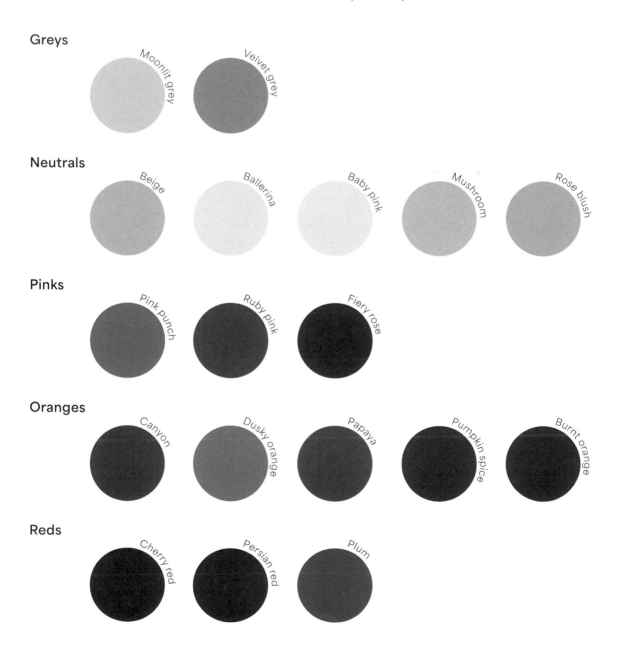

Greys

Moonlit grey

Velvet grey

Neutrals

Beige

Ballerina

Baby pink

Mushroom

Rose blush

Pinks

Pink punch

Ruby pink

Fiery rose

Oranges

Canyon

Dusky orange

Papaya

Pumpkin spice

Burnt orange

Reds

Cherry red

Persian red

Plum

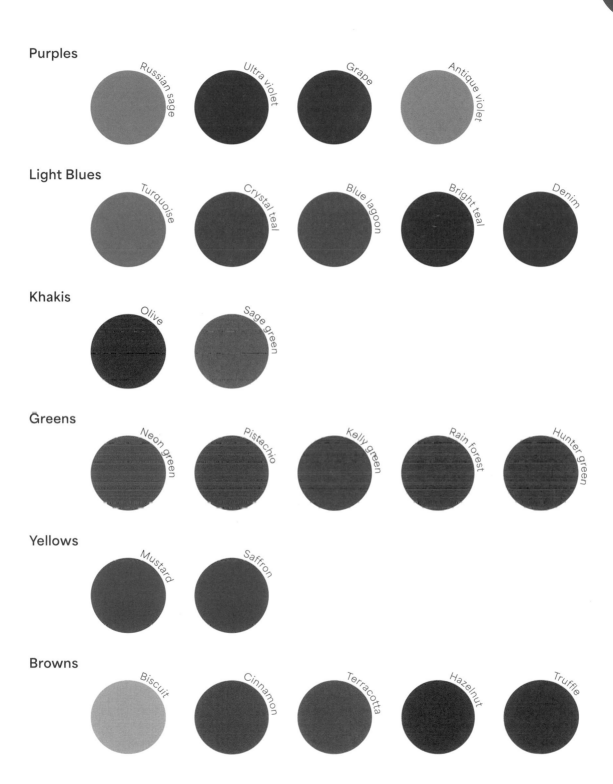

Purples

Russian sage   Ultra violet   Grape   Antique violet

Light Blues

Turquoise   Crystal teal   Blue lagoon   Bright teal   Denim

Khakis

Olive   Sage green

Greens

Neon green   Pistachio   Kelly green   Rain forest   Hunter green

Yellows

Mustard   Saffron

Browns

Biscuit   Cinnamon   Terracotta   Hazelnut   Truffle

The fresh face makeup palette

The guide below will help you to select the best makeup shades for your Lips, Eyes and Cheek to create a perfect everyday fresh face palette. I have included three depths of tones to every category: light, medium and deep. We have included Trinny London shades, but you can take this into any shop and match to the brand that you like.

Cool

Light

Lips
Maddie

Eyes
Mystery

Cheek
Pia

Medium

Lips
Bunny

Eyes
Wisdom

Cheek
Milly

Deep

Lips
Honor

Eyes
Joy

Cheek
Munchkin

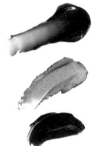

Cool/neutral

Light

Lips
Indi

Eyes
Justice

Cheek
Lady J

Medium

Lips
Bella

Eyes
Magician

Cheek
Phoebe

Deep

Lips
Freya

Eyes
Dawn

Cheek
Phoebe

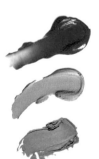

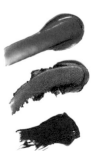

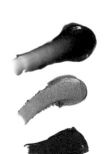

Neutral

Light

Lips
Dido

Eyes
Harmony

Cheek
Wiggs

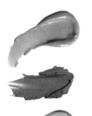

Medium

Lips
Cordy

Eyes
Dawn

Cheek
Reem

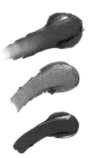

Deep

Lips
Bella

Eyes
Fortune

Cheek
Chloe

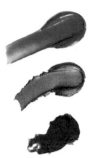

Warm/neutral

Light

Lips
Bella

Eyes
Virtue

Cheek
Veebee

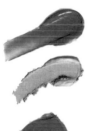

Medium

Lips
Emily

Eyes
Harmony

Cheek
Freddie

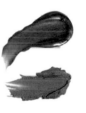

Deep

Lips
Lara

Eyes
Truth

Cheek
Freddie

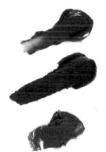

Warm

Light

Lips
Maiko

Eyes
Hope

Cheek
Sherin

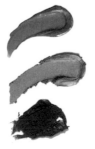

Medium

Lips
Lyla

Eyes
Fortune

Cheek
Rossy

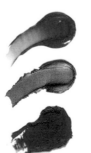

Deep

Lips
Weasie

Eyes
Empress

Cheek
Yassi

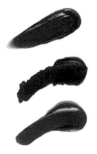

The statement lip makeup palette

The guide below will help you to select the best makeup shades for your Lips, Eyes and Cheek to create a palette for a fearless statement lip. I have included three depths of tones to every category: light, medium and deep. We have included Trinny London shades, but you can take this into any shop and match to the brand that you like.

Cool

Light

Lips
Demon

Eyes
Justice

Cheek
Katrin

Medium

Lips
Pippa

Eyes
Wisdom

Cheek
Schmoogie

Deep

Lips
Dalia

Eyes
Emperor

Cheek
Munchkin

Cool/neutral

Light

Lips
Valentina

Eyes
Virtue

Cheek
Electra

Medium

Lips
Pookie

Eyes
Magician

Cheek
Katrin

Deep

Lips
Demon

Eyes
Desire

Cheek
Yassi

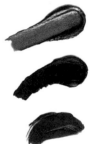
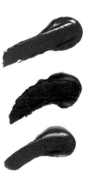

Neutral

Light

Lips
Pippa

Eyes
Dawn

Cheek
Lady J

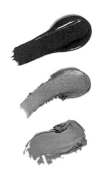

Medium

Lips
Demon

Eyes
Desire

Cheek
Reem

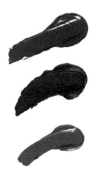

Deep

Lips
Pookie

Eyes
Empress

Cheek
Phoebe

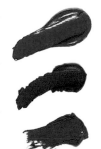

Warm/neutral

Light

Lips
Swainy

Eyes
Fortune

Cheek
Wiggs

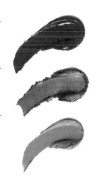

Medium

Lips
Valentina

Eyes
Trust

Cheek
Phoebe

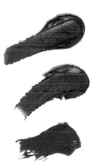

Deep

Lips
Valentina

Eyes
Emperor

Cheek
Yassi

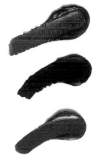

Warm

Light

Lips
Sacha

Eyes
Hope

Cheek
Sherin

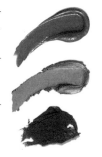

Medium

Lips
Katinka

Eyes
Harmony

Cheek
Freddie

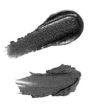

Deep

Lips
Swainy

Eyes
Fortune

Cheek
Chloe

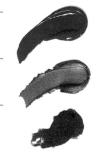

The smokey eye makeup palette

The guide below will help you to select the best makeup shades for your Lips, Eyes and Cheek to create a sultry smokey eye palette. I have included three depths of tones to every category: light, medium and deep. We have included Trinny London shades, but you can take this into any shop and match to the brand that you like.

Cool

Light

Lips
Dido

Eyes
Lovers

Cheek
Electra

Medium

Lips
Bunny

Eyes
Faith

Cheek
Schmoogie

Deep

Lips
Emily

Eyes
Strength

Cheek
Freddie

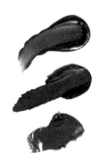

Cool/neutral

Light

Lips
Sooze

Eyes
Magician

Cheek
Lady J

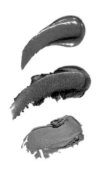

Medium

Lips
Bella

Eyes
Trust

Cheek
Phoebe

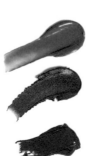

Deep

Lips
Weasie

Eyes
Desire

Cheek
Yassi

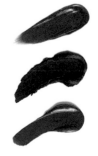

Neutral

Light

Lips
Eugenie

Eyes
Faith

Cheek
Schmoogie

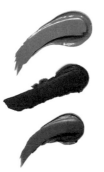

Medium

Lips
Emily

Eyes
Desire

Cheek
Freddie

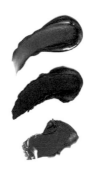

Deep

Lips
Thea

Eyes
Passion

Cheek
Munchkin

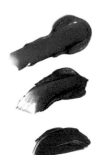

Warm/neutral

Light

Lips
Bella

Eyes
Trust

Cheek
Veebee

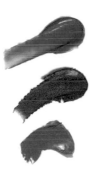

Medium

Lips
Katie

Eyes
Chariot

Cheek
Chloe

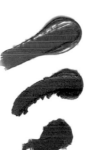

Deep

Lips
Bella

Eyes
Universe

Cheek
Freddie

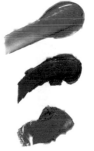

Warm

Light

Lips
Tashi

Eyes
Empress

Cheek
Wiggs

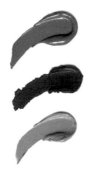

Medium

Lips
Weasie

Eyes
Empress

Cheek
Freddie

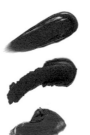

Deep

Lips
Aifric

Eyes
Queen

Cheek
Chloe

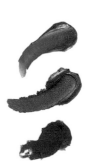

FEAR
LESS

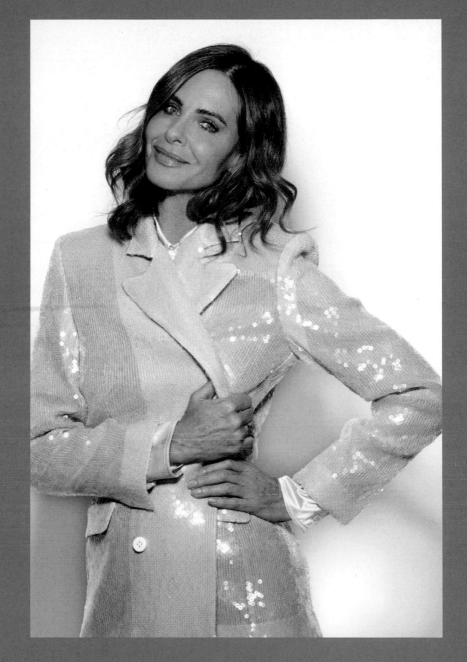

LIFE

FEEL INSPIRED

In this part I want you to feel energised and to learn new things.

I find joy in meeting people and hearing about their lives. I feel honoured when a woman trusts me enough to let me take her on a journey and reveals things about herself as part of the process. It gives me a sense of purpose, which is one of the ways that I fuel my energy.

In this section I cover the areas that have helped me to move forward in my life. These are here to act as inspiration and to provoke thoughts about where you are in your life right now. There's no rule, so if you try one and it doesn't work, that is fine - move on to something else.

Throughout this section and the rest of the book, I have included prompts where you will need to ask yourself questions (some easy and some hard) in order to challenge yourself in a variety of ways. I acknowledge that there is a big difference between reading and action, and it is the challenge to take action that will propel you to move forward. It will allow you to make positive changes in your own life and will give you the confidence to make decisions that are personal to your situation.

ENERGY UNDERPINS

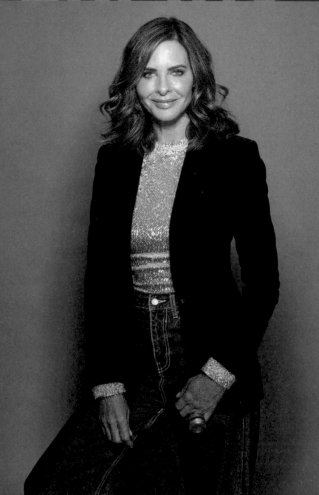

EVERYTHING WE DO

Supercharge your energy

Energy is the key to how we can move past our fear.

Being afraid saps our energy. It leads to stagnation, to feeling stuck in one place and unable to move forward. This can paralyse us and lower our confidence.

Perhaps you have a different word for it? You might call it life force or get-up-and-go. I think we all recognise that sunny-day feeling when we feel energised and ready to challenge ourselves. So much of what I want to talk about in these next pages comes down to this, to how we can grab hold of that feeling and get as much of it into our lives as possible.

When I do a Facebook or Instagram Live I have women that tune in and post comments and questions – that process of helping women makes me feel full of energy. If you can put energy out into the world, it will come back, like charging a battery.

What you wear promotes a certain energy. Consider a day where you might hide away in black versus when you step into some colour. Not only will it change your mood, but how those around you respond to you too.

Being afraid saps our energy

Self-worth & belief

Self-worth is believing that you are good enough and you deserve good things; it's about not putting yourself at the back of the queue. Self-belief is often drawn from times when you have faced a challenge and overcome it, big or small. It means having confidence in your abilities.

We can shy away from celebrating - or even acknowledging - the things we are good at because we worry it might come across as arrogance. When you have self-belief, you recognise what you can do and what you know, and it gives you the energy to strive to learn about the things you don't. We have to actively nurture both **self-worth** and **self-belief** because they help us to deal with our fears.

Self-acceptance comes with an implicit flip side: that you accept the way things are and you don't have the power to change them. What we want is clarity and purpose - to see and like ourselves for who we are and to be the best version of that. For example, if you feel you are disorganised, or you can be overly critical, or you aren't looking after your health properly, you don't need to accept that as a given if it is making you unhappy.

We have to actively nurture self-worth and self-belief

Imposter syndrome limits us

I feel like now is a good time for a word about imposter syndrome. While I recognise the feeling I do wonder if this is a useful term to be using. Doesn't it feel very weighty? Almost like an illness. 'I can't do that, I have imposter syndrome.'

Labels weigh us down. If you don't feel like you should be in the room, what do you need to believe that you do? If it's more knowledge, can you find someone who can help you with that? If it's more experience, well, you are only going to get that if you are in that room! Women can feel like imposters if they don't think they know 90 per cent of what is going on. But that's rarely the case. And usually someone has invited you or encouraged you into that space in the first place. Do you trust their opinion? They clearly value your contribution.

'Imposter syndrome' is a good example of a time when we look at others' exteriors, to the confident face they present to the world, and compare it to our fearful interior. Other people feel insecure too, you just can't always see it. It is also an opportunity to use common sense to talk back to the negative voice in our head and accept that it is what it is. It can be a part of us that occasionally likes to get overly loud. I always used to tell it to quieten down, but recently realised that this might be a version of our younger self that needs kinder words and reassurance from our older selves in order to keep moving forward positively.

You need to value your contribution

You are not your thoughts

This can be so incredibly difficult to do when you are struggling but finding a way to separate your thoughts from yourself, to recognise them as just thoughts and not intrinsic to who you are, is such an important thing.

When I was 24 I went to rehab. After five months there, I went to live in a halfway house in Weston-Super-Mare for another seven months. When I eventually got back to London, everything was completely overwhelming. I felt stripped raw. I walked down my local street and I had a panic attack.

In rehab I learned to recognise dark thoughts as something that were separate to me. I imagined them as a black raven squawking in my ear. I didn't have to put up with it, though – with practice, I could turn to this debilitating, annoying bird and tell it to shut up. I learnt to tell myself, 'This is not me, this is one thought inside my head that has a lot of thoughts, a lot of things going on. Tomorrow I could wake up feeling different because thoughts change – I can change them.' Some days that worked better than others, but after a while the black raven got quieter and quieter.

The other thing to remember is that fear and negative thoughts fester in the dark. When you shine a light on them they often feel less overwhelming. You can see them for what they are and begin to find a way to process them. When we feel low or not ourselves it's tempting to shut ourselves away from others. We might feel like no one else understands, like we don't know how to explain how we feel or simply that we are not very good company so our friends won't want to hear from us. But it is so important to reach out. Those around you can help you if you let them.

It's important to be aware of any negative thought patterns. It is worth considering a form of therapy, app or helpline if you find they are debilitating or you are struggling. I have been to therapy in my life and there are many types you can try. Do reach out. Traditional therapy can be expensive, so I have left some details at the end for other places you can reach out to (see page 348).

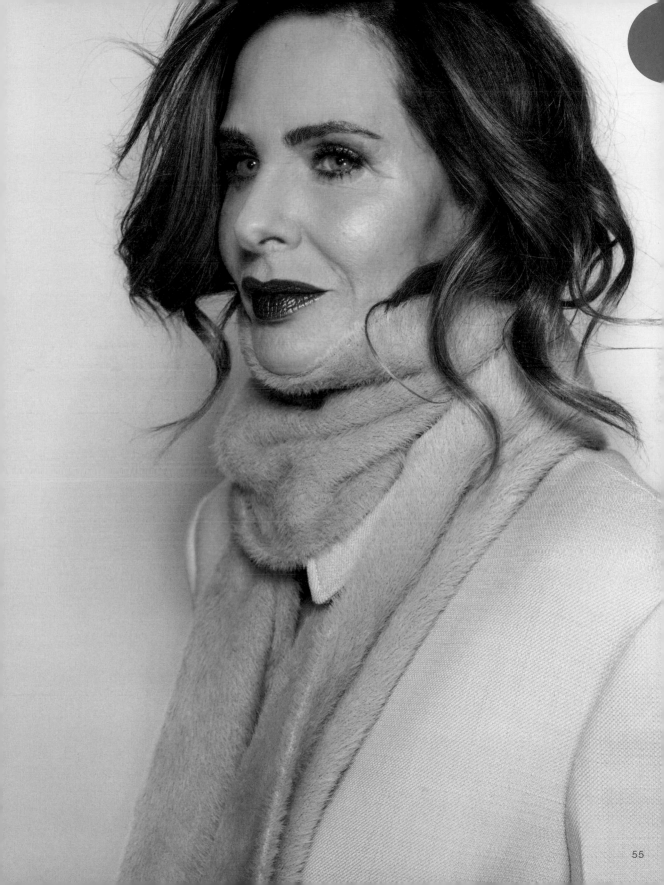

55

ASK YOURSELF

1   Do you feel you are low in confidence?

2   Do you nurture your self-worth when you feel low?

3   Do you always put other people's needs before your own?

4   Do you ever say no?

5   Do you struggle to feel present in the room?

6   Do you feel your contributions to the room are welcome?

7   Do you struggle with self-belief?

8   Do you have a strategy for coping with negative thoughts?

CHALLENGE YOURSELF

Loneliness and tiredness

Isolation and tiredness are very corroding to self-worth. Sometimes we forget who our friends are and think we can't call, but always reach out and remember that if the roles were reversed, you would take that call. Also consider saying no to those who drain you and consciously take time for yourself.

Self-belief

Quite a lot of self-belief is attached to other people's belief in us. We can challenge ourselves by showing others we believe in ourselves, even through a 'fake it to make it' mentality. The more we believe, the more others will too. When Susannah and I had a column in the *Telegraph* we felt we deserved a pay rise, but it was difficult to ask for one. I read over letters from our readers telling us how much what we wrote meant to them. This reminded me that not only did I love the work but it was of value to other people too. I rode the resultant wave right into the editor's office and we got what we asked for! Have confidence in your own experience and find a mentor who can help with any gaps.

Remember who you really are

Do this when you are feeling good so you have it in place for times when you are not. Think of the positive things that people would say about you and, unashamedly, write them down. You need to be reminded of how fabulous other people think you are when you do not feel it yourself.

A gratitude list

I have done this for years, and it can be very simple. Write down what you are grateful for - a roof over your head, a job you love ...

Intuition & instinct are different

The words instinct and intuition are often used interchangeably but to me they are two very different things. My instinct isn't always correct but I should always follow my intuition.

Instinct can come from a place of fear. It is connected to the fight/flight/freeze impulse that is hardwired into our animal brains. Your instinct is to avoid things that have the power to hurt you.

Intuition, however, is deeper than this. It comes from all your experiences, your innate sense of what is right for you. It's not always an immediate reaction - sometimes you can only follow your intuition when a question has percolated in your brain, when you have allowed reason and logic to sit alongside an emotional reaction.

Generally speaking, I think instinct leads you to defend your position whereas listening to your intuition encourages you to be brave. Instinct tells you 'be careful, this is risky'; intuition says 'I can do this. This is worth a try.

It's so important to own the decision. The hardest thing is often making a decision and getting ready to make that leap. It's very freeing when you have done it. It takes a lot of energy to be constantly deliberating. It's exhausting. When you know what you are going to do your mindset changes. It builds your sense of self when you make difficult decisions. We can never be sure of the outcome but we can cultivate faith in our power to choose a course of action.

Intuition encourages you to be brave

ASK YOURSELF

1   Do you recognise the difference between instinct and intuition?

2   When you made a bad decision recently or in your past, what was driving you?

3   Are your decisions driven by the fear you feel about the possible outcomes?

4   Is there anything in your life now that is holding you back from where you want to go?

CHALLENGE YOURSELF

Write it down

In times of uncertainty, it can be helpful to jot down your feelings surrounding a situation. What do you recognise as coming from an instinct to protect yourself, to stay where it feels safe? And what is your intuition telling you that you want, what opportunities lie ahead? You can sort these feelings into two lists – instinct and intuition. What feels more powerful, most persuasive to you?

Standing on quicksand or solid ground

There are times when fear becomes an engine driving us to change. This is when we reach a point where we are too scared to carry on as we are. The fear of nothing changing outweighs the fear of making the change.

It was this feeling that made me drive myself to rehab. I had been scared of being without the social insulation of drugs because I was shy and I didn't know myself, though I didn't understand it as this at the time. But I became scared of how little I had begun to care, how detached I was from my emotions. I used to have passion and joie de vivre and drive but I realised I had lost it all. I had become more afraid of not stopping than I was of the implications of giving up.

After I got clean I moved back home aged 27. My friends' lives had carried on while I was away; I felt they were far ahead of me, with good jobs, earning money, while I was starting over. Without drugs, I had nothing to hide behind. I felt like I was living on quicksand.

One of the mantras of Alcoholics Anonymous (AA) is 'one day at a time'. You deal only with what is right in front of you, rather than panicking about a bigger picture over which you don't feel in control. You give yourself a horizon that is right in front of your nose and you keep the learning curves small. Then, as you reach milestones and achieve simple goals, you broaden your horizons.

Fear can drive you to make the biggest changes in your life, even if it is a difficult and painful place to be. Fear can be fuel. It's almost like we can burn through it to move on and be free. It was fear that kept me clean once out of rehab. Three of my closest friends decided to get clean when I did, but I was the only one who went through with it. Heartbreakingly, within two years, they had all died.

After taking it 'one day at a time', my horizon did begin to broaden. Small things helped me rebuild my confidence and the future felt like something to look forward to rather than fear. I no longer feel like I am living on quicksand. Now, when faced with a future fear, I have more tools to work through it and I can land on solid ground.

ASK YOURSELF

1   Do you use anything that gives you social insulation?
          Or use alcohol or drugs as a social crutch?

2   Are you always questioning your decisions?

3   Do you feel stuck?

4   Do you feel a mixture of very emotional
          and quite detached?

CHALLENGE YOURSELF

Test any dependency

If you answered yes to question 1, challenge yourself to
abstain for a week or longer. Check in with how you are
feeling and, if you need to, seek professional help.

Write a journal

Consider doing this every morning and write what you want
to do today. Don't think about tomorrow, and only include
things that are achievable (not climbing Everest!). It will fuel
your self-worth to accomplish your plans for the day.

Notice your feelings

Try to get through a day without feeling either envy or
pity. These feelings make us unsettled. If you do feel
them, try to write down why you do, so that you can
better understand the feeling and put it in perspective.

The art of letting go

As humans, we crave control. We want to know that if we put the work in we will get the result we want. We want to be sure of outcomes and it makes us hold tight to things in a bid to avoid feeling like they are out of our hands. But sometimes we have to let go.

There are different kinds of letting go.

There are times when you have given something your all and you have to let the ship sail and see what comes back.

Then there are situations in which we have let go of some control so others can grow. Perhaps you can be a micromanager at work and you need to step back and allow others in your team to make decisions. Or you have a teenager who wants more freedom and you have to believe that you have brought them up well enough that they can start to make their own choices, away from your supervision.

And then there is the letting go of the small things that have little impact on where you want to get to but that are drawing your focus and holding you back. This version of letting go is about zooming out to see the big picture so you can recognise what is draining the energy that can be better spent elsewhere.

The hardest kind of letting go is when you have been striving for something that has felt incredibly important but for some reason it has not worked out how you expected. A relationship, a goal, a milestone, a dream.

I have had to do this a few times in my life and it is always painful. In the late 1990s, I set up an internet startup that didn't work out. Closing that business – something that many people had put so much work into – really made me question my ability.

But possibly the hardest was when I had to give up my dream home. After I split up with my husband I became determined to buy somewhere on this particular street that I always walked past when taking Lyla to school. So I borrowed money, I got a large mortgage and really over extended myself to buy this house and do it up. I took it apart and rebuilt it and I was so proud of the result. It was something tangible and totally mine, for the first time ever, which felt like a big moment. But I'd done it in a way that wasn't secure.

Just a year after I moved in, I realised that I was too stretched. I cut back and tried to rearrange my finances but it was still strained. My ex-husband then died, which brought further financial complications. I also wanted to set up my new business, Trinny London. I had a moment of clarity when I saw that in order to build something with real potential, I was going to have to give up the thing I had wanted the most – that house. I had to let it go. It was more important to be debt free and renting, than own a home with great financial burden. I would worry so much about the finances, I would not be able to focus on making my business a success, which was my bigger future.

The thing about letting go is that while it can feel very frightening to cast off a big focus in your life, perhaps something that even feels a part of who you are, It opens up space for other things to come in. A few months after I closed our startup, Susannah and I were asked to do *What Not to Wear* by the BBC. Moving out of that home made it possible to set up Trinny London – something I am so proud of and which brings me so much joy and fulfilment.

It's easier to let go when you can see what that will open up for you in another area. It makes it possible to see letting go as a positive thing, rather than an absence or a loss. Though it's still hard, particularly when you are emotionally invested or you fear a lack of control. Examining the evidence and looking objectively at what you need, what you value and what is either adding to your life or sticking you to one place is important here. Sometimes you have to jump and have faith that the landing will be OK, there will be a net, even if you don't see it at first glance.

Facing the unknown

We want to feel certain of outcomes because we have a natural fear of the unknown. Living with uncertainty is incredibly hard. It feels uncomfortable and can require all of our reserves of resilience and self-belief.

The most profound experience I have had of this in my life was when I was going through IVF. If you have done IVF then you will know the feeling of having to keep faith in the process while dealing with the uncertainty as to whether it will turn out the way you want. Each cycle comes with intense hope and the potential for intense disappointment.

My relationship with my mother was a complicated one and I questioned whether I would be a good mother. I had no burning desire to be a parent until I hit 35. But then it didn't happen, and so we went down the route of IVF. Round after round didn't work. I did three a year for over three years.

I lived through times of thinking I would never have a child but simultaneously never truly giving up. My intuition told me I was going to be a mother in some capacity - it could have been that energy would go into being a good step-mother to my step-son or some other way. I felt I wanted to mother a child and that I would, somehow.

But it still wasn't working. IVF puts a strain on your relationships and on all other areas of your life. I got pregnant twice, but lost both babies. I started to let go of the concept of having a child and thought maybe what I was doing wasn't the right thing. But then I became pregnant with Lyla. The joy was of course accompanied by the continual underlying fear that I would lose the baby. I had a scan every two weeks and I had to live with a different type of uncertainty in a situation I was powerless to control.

That whole journey taught me something important about fear. Sometimes I managed it really well and sometimes I didn't. There was certainly an element of narrowing my horizons again, of dealing primarily with what was right in front of me to try to cope with the crashing waves of 'What if...?' To continually live in that abyss of uncertainty I had to find ways of letting go and releasing some of the fear.

I did IVF again after I had Lyla but I gave up after five more rounds. I had my little girl and I let go of the possibility of having another child.

We all want to write the ending we dream of, but you can't. Finding a way to live with life's big unknowns teaches us resilience. Facing them head on one day at a time helps us find ways to manage our fear and move forward.

You might be facing a similar challenge right now. And all I know is that the more we hold onto something, the less we can see a different outcome. This alternate outcome has the potential to bring just as much happiness, but we are not able to imagine it. The thing is, we don't know what is behind the closed door and it might be even more glorious.

You never know what is behind the closed door, it might be even more glorious

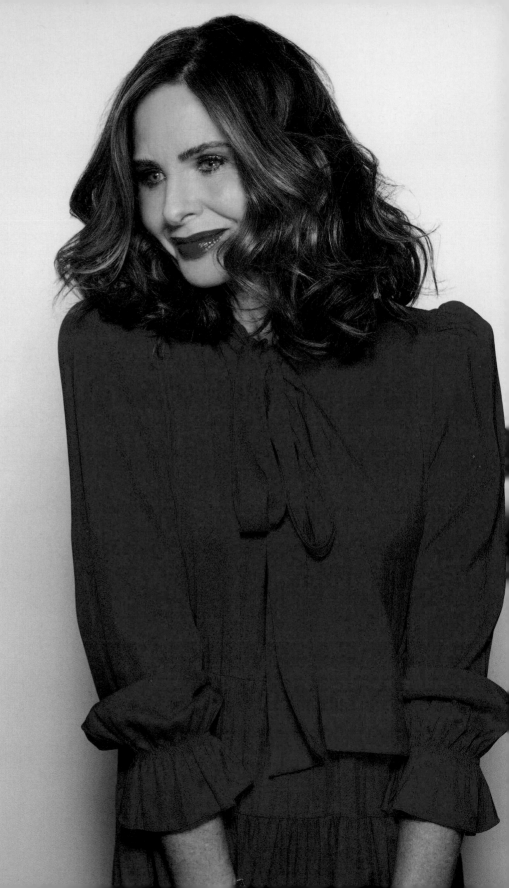

Setting your intentions

I always want to feel like I am living in a moving current. Sometimes I am swimming against it and sometimes it's carrying me along in the direction I want to go. That sense of movement, of going somewhere, gives me energy.

In either of these instances, I need a lighthouse to guide me. I need the beams to give me self-motivation, otherwise I am swimming without an aim.

Do you set New Year's resolutions? I do reflect and set intentions in January, but I find September is a better time of year for me to stop and consider the big picture. If you grew up in the northern hemisphere you might still get that September back-to-school feeling, hard-wired from the new academic year beginning at the end of the summer. Also, when Susannah and I were making our television shows, it was always in September that we would find out if we were going to be recommissioned for another series. The narrative around January resolutions can focus on your personal motivational improvements, whereas in September it feels easier to ask 'what do I want to do next?' – which is a far healthier and more productive question for that time of year.

It doesn't matter what time of year works for your internal rhythm as long as you do find time to pause and think about the next stage of your journey and ask if all the elements of your life are still working for the person you are now.

It's not just an annual thing. Do you take time to regularly check in, to set intentions and think about your goals? I'm not just talking about the big milestones, like a step up in your career or moving house. Are you spending enough time with your friends? Are you nurturing your body with the right food, enough sleep and exercise? If you really want to start something new but you keep putting it off, why is that?

I get knocked down, but I get up again

Perseverance means putting one foot in front of the other. It is doggedly getting back up when you are knocked down rather than lying on the ground until someone comes to help you.

Tenacity is more proactive, more creative. It is about facing adversity and uncertainty and looking for opportunities, for gaps you can squeeze through or possible advantages. For this you need energy. For perseverance, you just need to not stop.

There are times in all of our lives when all we can do is persevere as best we can. And there are times when we need to look up from the slow plod of our feet against the prevailing wind and scan the wider horizon for possibilities.

Confidence, self-belief, self-esteem and tenacity are like an ecosystem, they all feed each other. When we practise or nurture one, it grows the others.

There are definitely times when my energy is low and I need to take a duvet therapy day. That's absolutely fine. The key is to know when it's time to get back up again and to tune into opportunities as they come up.

I think it is helpful to have both perseverance and tenacity, but do you identify with one more than the other and can you make sure there is balance in your life?

The key is to know when it's time to get back up

The 99 per cent

'99 per cent of everything you worry about never happens, Trinny.'

This is something my husband Johnny used to say to me. And I would say it to Lyla: 'Remember what Dadda says – 99 per cent of everything you worry about never happens.'

Of course, the 1 per cent did happen to us. We lost Johnny.

But I still say it to myself because it's true. There's an expression I heard once that worrying is like paying interest on a debt you don't owe. It is a needless expenditure of energy on things that aren't worth it because they are unlikely to happen. And when they do, well, that is out of our control.

I had to deal with the terrible fallout of Johnny's death and Lyla has had to grow up without her dad. But we are still here; we are still standing and she is thriving.

Resilience is an interesting word. An old-fashioned understanding of it is to keep going regardless, without stopping to acknowledge or talk about what has hurt you. But it is as unhelpful to ignore your emotions as it is to absorb negativity, letting every worry and setback get to you.

I think resilience is linked to tenacity. It's about building confidence and self-belief so you can keep moving forward on a motivated journey to wherever it is you want to go. Bad things will happen, and you will stay strong and keep going. Ninety-nine per cent of the things you worry about won't happen. But the fear will sap your energy and keep you stuck. For me, the sense of freedom that comes from conquering fear is one of the best feelings there is.

The quadrants tool

When we are deciding what we want to bring into our lives it is so useful to understand where we are right now. Perhaps you need to let something go to make space for something you want?

You may well be familiar with this technique. Its real name is a 'time management matrix' but I think of it as 'the quadrants'. It's a simple and flexible tool that can bring clarity as it allows us to reflect on how we spend our time and what we see as important.

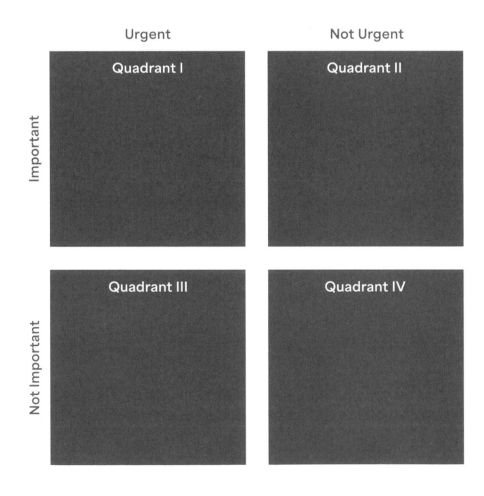

	Urgent	Not Urgent
Important	Quadrant I	Quadrant II
Not Important	Quadrant III	Quadrant IV

How to use the quadrants tool

What tasks do you have right now that are urgent and important? These are the things you need to do soon or there will be undesirable consequences. This can be anything from filing a tax return, to making time to go for a daily walk, because it's important for your mental health. Some of these things will be unavoidable 'life admin' and some will be more specific to you. Put these in the top left-hand box. Many of these start off as important and not urgent, but as they aren't dealt with they tip over into another box.

Now think about what is important to you but does not have a pressing deadline. Perhaps this is going on holiday, decorating a room in your house, organising to see your friends or something you want to focus more on at work. Add these things to the top right-hand box.

In the bottom left-hand box put tasks that you feel need your attention but the consequences of not getting to them are less significant. Household chores may fall into this category as well as more minor tasks that come with a deadline.

The bottom right-hand box will prompt you to think about the things you spend time on that are not important and not urgent. How much of your week is given over to things inside this box? How can you divide your day in a more constructive way? This will increase your self-worth and give you a sense of achievement.

When filling in the quadrants, areas to consider are:

- Commitments to family

- Work and career

- Relationships (romantic and with friends)

- Home

- Planning holidays

- Self-development/spiritual

- Self-care

ASK YOURSELF

1 Is everything in the right box?

2 How have you decided what is important and what is less so?

3 How can you minimise the things that are not urgent and not important?

4 Are there any individual tasks that have been in the 'urgent and important' category for a while?

5 What do you really mean when you say 'I haven't got time'?

CHALLENGE YOURSELF

The meaning of urgency

What would happen if the things you see as urgent and important weren't done? Alternatively, does anything need elevating so you give it more attention? For example, if you don't see your friends you may feel lonely, in which case that becomes more urgent.

Priorities

Do you decide what is important or are you responding to pressure from others? Unless they are your boss, you do not have to make someone else's urgency your urgency all of the time.

The small things

Can you remove any of the tasks or elements that are not urgent or not important? Try to clear off tasks that could be done quickly.

Time

If this is your reason for not having tackled something that is urgent or important, interrogate this further. Is it this simple, or are you putting it off for another reason? Is it really urgent? Is it important to you or is it pressure from elsewhere that makes you feel you should see it that way? Is this something you could remove from your life to free up energy better spent elsewhere?

You decide what is important

When you have more clarity about what you need to do and what is important to you, you can create space to allow you more focus. You will have a greater understanding of what your priorities actually are and you can move forward with greater intentionality and give importance to the things that nurture you too.

Set yourself goals for now

Every year, I like to set myself around 10 goals to work towards over the course of the next 12 months. They will not all necessarily look like big achievements from the outside - the most important thing is that they matter to me.

When setting goals, I think there should be a balance between the emotional things and the material or practical things that you want to bring into your life. An emotional goal might be feeling better about your body, nurturing a relationship, growing your confidence at work. Practical goals tend to be more straightforward, for example, decluttering, finding an exercise class you enjoy and will stick to, being more organised. A material goal might be to buy a new car or move house.

I do think when you focus too much on a financial gain, however, it doesn't create good energy. It can make you feel fear because it involves putting a certain value on what you deem to be success. So while financial goals are important - we all want to feel financially stable and money is a fact of life - they shouldn't pull all of our focus.

Don't be afraid to set a goal even if you don't initially know how you will make it happen. If you really want it you will find a way. You can break it into stages, find people to help you, learn a skill to get you there. Set the goal and challenge yourself to make a plan.

When we think about a goal, we can focus too much on the outcome - the finish line, the celebration when we get there. We also need to think about what the journey there will be like.

If you are pushing yourself to do something new, there will almost certainly be steps on the way that are challenging. If you don't imagine them and what they might feel like, it increases their potential power to derail you. For example, if you want to run a marathon you may decide to train first thing in the morning. So how are you going to motivate yourself to get out of bed when it's cold? What will you need to keep going on days when it feels particularly hard?

Imagination is such a powerful thing. We can't do anything unless we can imagine it first. So imagine practical and emotional challenges of the journey too, as well as visualising the outcome, and it will help you to get there. You can put it on a moodboard so that it visually exists too.

It also comes back to energy. What is going to give you the energy, the fuel in your engine, to carry you along that road? Don't think it's going to come out of thin air somehow. It won't. Energy can be an incredibly motivating friend who checks in with you; looking after your body so you feel good; introducing a new exercise into your routine so you have stamina; space to think a decision through and feel excited – these are all really important.

The final thing I want to say about goals is to always check in to make sure they are truly yours. We can all feel pressure to tick boxes and reach milestones by certain points in our lives. If you haven't and you compare yourself to friends who have, it can leave you feeling down on yourself or lacking confidence. But are these goals right for you? I used to talk about how I didn't own my home; it felt significant because it is something you are 'supposed' to aim for. But now I am changing that narrative about myself because I see that I have taken a different path.

Some people's identities get caught up with where they 'should be' at certain points. It is a very human thing to compare ourselves to others. But this can cloud our judgement and get in the way of going after what we really want.

Challenge yourself to make a plan

How to set intention

I like to choose a word of the month. It might be two words, or it may be a phrase. It is different to a goal as it is about grounding me in what I want to hold close to me that month. It is usually connected to what is happening in my life at the time. It might come from wanting to be present, to remember to take time for myself, to enjoy the journey. I don't put a lot of conscious thought into what they should be; my intuition tells me what is right.

For example:

- Listen and learn

- Clarity and sensation

- Feel the fear and do it anyway

I have a set intention. There are so many demands on our time and attention I find that setting an intention brings focus to one small area I care about. For example, I recently decided not to shop for a month. That's a practical thing, but more than that I wanted to identify why I shop and how I can sometimes replace that urge to buy with other positive things.

Write or print out your word of the month and your intention and put them somewhere you will see them every day, as a reminder. For example, above the kettle so it catches your eye while you're making a cup of tea. Or on your mirror in the bedroom so you see them first thing in the morning. I put mine on my laptop.

If you are a very visual person, perhaps an image or a photo will inspire you and remind you of an intention. When I was setting up Trinny London, I had a fabulous photo of the pioneering female pilot Amelia Earhart putting on her lipstick in the cockpit of a plane. The glamour and the spirit of adventure that picture encapsulates really spoke to me at the time.

The wonders of meditation

I find meditation and visioning useful for so many reasons. It brings me clarity, it renews my energy and it clears my head of a tremendous amount of noise. It also helps me to deal with stress.

Stress can keep us stuck in a place where we can't focus on anything else other than the source of our stress. I find that it affects my memory and focus, and meditation is a great way to manage this.

There is almost an infinite number of types of meditation – it is such an umbrella term. For some people, it is a very spiritual practice – this is where it originated, after all. But don't let that intimidate you if you have yet to try it. It doesn't have to be complicated and it can be used as a tool in your life in many different ways. You may feel like you will struggle to 'clear you mind' but it is not always about this.

I did some meditation when I was fundraising for Trinny London that comes under the category of 'visioning'. I imagined the products being made on the factory floor, then being packed up in boxes and going around the world, eventually being opened by women who I hoped would get joy from them. This kind of exercise is about harnessing the power of imagination. It made me feel very focused and energised.

I have been very fortunate to meet some amazing experts and specialists who have taught me a great deal about their fields and I am going to introduce you to some of them in the next few pages so they can share some of their wisdom with you too. Jo Bowlby (who has a brilliant book called *A Book for Life*) and Sanjai Verma are two practitioners who have helped me with meditation practices, and the exercises that follow have come to me from them.

Harness the power of your imagination

A meditation exercise for stress and anxiety

The 'five senses' meditation is a simple way of bringing your focus into the moment and slowing a racing brain. I do it a lot when I'm on a train of thought I can't get off. It's a well-known technique as it is very effective and you can do it anywhere at any time.

Start with a few good, deep breaths. Look around you and consciously notice five things that you can see. Try to really take in the colours, shapes and small details of these things.

Now you can close your eyes if you want to. Try to notice four things around you that you can hear. It may be the sound of your own breathing, traffic, conversation. Take a moment to focus on each of those four things.

What can you feel? This can be anything from the texture of the clothes on your body to the sensation of your feet on the floor to how you are feeling inside. How do you feel sitting in this still state?

Now think about what you can smell. Try to pick up on two distinct smells. And finally, what can you taste? Is there a taste currently in your mouth that you can identify and name?

When you have done this, you can take a deep breath and release the focus.

A visioning technique when someone is dominating or diminishing you

This is so useful if there is someone in your life who is making you feel small or like they are taking away some of your power and energy and you need to reduce their impact on you.

You can do this in the moment when the person is sitting in front of you or you can imagine that they are. Think about them getting smaller and smaller. Imagine their feet dangling, getting further away from the floor as they shrink down, until they look like a small doll taking up hardly any space in the middle of the chair. In your mind's eye, look down on their small form and think about how much bigger you are by comparison.

A meditation exercise for energy

We are made from atoms, which contain positive and negative charge. Even when we feel depleted or exhausted we contain energy and this exercise is a way to physically feel that energy within us and channel it.

Sit down, get comfortable and take a few slow breaths. With your elbows at your sides raise your hands straight in front of you with your palms facing. Close your eyes if you want to and focus on feeling a sense of energy between your palms. If you really concentrate you may feel your fingers start to tingle. Imagine what this ball of energy might look like and move your hands around it. Try slowly moving your hands apart to see if you can grow the energy between them. Now push them closer together to really compact that ball of energy. When you are ready, push that energy into your chest with your hands, shoving it into your heart.

It is time to exercise

When I was younger I hated exercise so much that I faked a bad cough consistently for years so I could get out of playing sport at school. Running around a pitch in the rain or swimming in the freezing cold did not appeal.

When I was about 23 I started doing Pilates – I think it was the grace of it and its association with ballet dancers that made me try it. I have never liked things that make me sweat, although when I was 35 I did take up boxing for a while, training with a guy who had been a champion boxer. It appealed partly because of the mental side – it involved skills I could learn.

I now know how important exercise is. Seeing my mother slow down as she got older had a big impact on me. She suffered from swollen knees and as a result, she didn't do much exercise as she got older, which made walking much harder for her. It made me very aware that I wanted to use exercise as a way to be as mobile as possible for as long as possible.

The value of exercise for mental health is widely discussed now, as well as the health dangers of having a sedentary lifestyle. Though I do think that can feel dispiriting if you have never enjoyed exercise, if you feel you are starting from a place of low fitness or if you are lacking in body confidence. The main thing is to choose a form of exercise you enjoy – or can at least bear to do – and find a way to stick with it. Recognise what motivates you. Does being outdoors make you feel good? Are you more likely to go to a class where there is a social aspect, at a set time every week? Does it help to listen to music or podcasts when you work out?

What you wear to work out may seem like a minor detail but it is important. If you put on something old and shapeless it will reinforce any belief you have that this is not something you want to be doing, that it's not for you. Instead, find some leggings in a fun pattern or a great colour that you actually want to put on. Try to wear fitted workout clothes – if you don't like the lumps and bumps then choose a thick fabric designed to support you. You will notice the changes to your body quicker and feel more energised.

If you feel self-conscious exercising, remember no one is looking at you. The other people in the gym or the class are far more worried about what they are doing.

I really would urge every woman to consider some form of strength training. It is one of the most important things you can do to keep you mobile and active as you go down the path of life and it is never too early or late to start. Not only does it improve your balance and stability, it increases bone density, which is vital for protecting against osteoporosis. Plus there is something very satisfying about picking up a heavy box and realising you are quite capable of moving it by yourself.

Nowadays, alongside strength training, I walk, I do yoga and I still do Pilates. I see it as a necessity. I don't love it every time and I often feel like cancelling, but I know I will feel so happy when I have done it. Whatever you do, do something. Start somewhere. Focus on what you can do – not what you feel you can't – and build from there. Love yourself enough to invest in your body and take the time to exercise.

Yoga

Victoria Woodhall started teaching me yoga in September 2020. Before this, I had been put off by the idea you had to spend a long time learning complicated poses and treat it all with great reverence. Of course, you can do this if you want, but Victoria's approach is about getting stronger, good balance (so important as we go down the path of life), breathwork and stretching out all those muscles that get scrunched up when we hunch over a desk all day. In her words, it all comes down to 'moving and breathing'.

If you are already sold on all the benefits of yoga you have my permission to skip this bit. If you are on the fence, then I will step aside and let Victoria try to convince you herself …

Why practise yoga
by Victoria Woodhall

Yoga is a practice that meets you where you are, at whatever life stage, and develops and changes with you, carrying you forwards, onwards and upwards.

It's often thought that yoga is all about being flexible, and for many people that's not just a turn-off but a barrier to entry: 'I can't touch my toes, therefore this is not for me.' Unless you have ambitions to join the circus, let that misconception go – and give yoga a try.

It's one of the best all-round practices for strength, stability and balance in body and mind – all valuable life skills in a world where so much can knock us off course. Yes, flexibility will come, but it's not the goal. Yoga gives you endless ways to feel better, to get stronger, experience your full range of motion, to try new challenges and feel more confident in what you can do as you get older. Who says you can't learn to do a headstand in your fifties? My father nailed crow pose – a fun arm balance – on his seventy-ninth birthday. Now that's fearless!

Yoga puts a spring in our step and makes us feel lighter. Lengthening, strengthening and coordinating our muscles means we can move through life with ease and fluidity, comfortable in our own skin and youthful in the way we carry ourselves.

Because yoga is also a breathing practice – we move in time with the steady rhythm of the breath, like dancing to our own beat – it can have powerful and immediate mental and emotional benefits, which is often the reason why people say they feel better after class. By focusing on a steady breath we can calm the minds chatter and turn down the volume on the inner critic that so loves to hold us back.

Just as there are many styles of music, there are hundreds of styles of yoga and yoga teachers and it's important to find the one that suits you. Above all, it should make you feel so good that you want to come back. Be prepared to try a few before you find your 'fit'. But once you do, you'll enjoy the journey of 'you' that much more.

Our relationship with sugar

Eating the right things is one of the most important ways we nurture our bodies. Whatever size your body, whatever it can or can't do, it is yours and it deserves to be taken care of, inside and out.

If we feel sluggish and tired, a lack of nutrients is so often at least part of the cause. Learning to listen to our body and what it is actually asking for is key. When we are tired or sad it is so easy to reach for chocolate or cake to make us feel better. When we are swamped with work or family commitments, ready-made processed food feels so convenient. We all do it from time to time and it's important not to let feelings of shame in here, but also to recognise that we are not doing ourselves any favours longterm.

Problems arise if the messages our body is sending us get scrambled. For example, if you automatically reach for a sugary snack when you are exhausted, your body will become used to this and is more likely to crave sugar, which is a cause of inflammation in the body. When what it really wants is rest, perhaps more nutrients, even to wake up and move around.

Since the menopause, I really notice when I have anything containing a significant amount of sugar. I feel the inflammation it causes, particularly in my ankles. Which does make me stop and consider what else it might be doing to my body.

If you are someone who eats a lot of sugar, consider trying to give it up for a few of weeks. You may experience side effects – some people report sleeplessness, irritability, cravings and headaches – such is the impact of sugar on our bodies, so make sure you do your research first so you know what to expect. This can be a really good way to reset your relationship with sugar and show yourself that you don't need to reach for snacks and treats that aren't doing you any good.

The pitfalls of alcohol

That alcohol is not good for you is not headline news. But we can become complacent in our relationship with alcohol and put up with the sluggishness, dull skin, poor sleep and mild depression and anxiety it increasingly brings.

For some, alcohol feels like a useful shortcut - to feeling relaxed or more sociable at the end of a stressful day. Our relationship to alcohol can also be quite emotional and we fear change: you might worry how your girlfriends will react if you turn down the customary gin and tonics on holiday or what your partner will say if you decline to open a nice bottle of red to go with a dinner they have made you. But it's important to focus on yourself here. It is not worth compromising on your health and your energy levels for the sake of anyone else's opinion.

Alcohol becomes bad for you when you begin to feel more depressed, when you feel inflammation in your body and when you can't get through a difficult situation without it. Of course it can be wonderfully social, but you should worry if it starts to compromise your health or your energy levels. You might be the kind of person who feels under pressure to drink, but another sign of really taking care of yourself is being able to say no. If you can't do that easily, ask yourself why.

If you are giving up alcohol, you will probably crave a lot of sugar. I am not trying to be a killjoy, but any extra sugar will make you feel sluggish and cause inflammation in the body, undoing some of the good work you have done avoiding the booze, thereby making you less likely to persevere. It will become a vicious cycle.

If you are worried you have a problem with alcohol, there are many ways to get help. You could go to a newcomers meeting at AA, where you might be really suprised by the feeling of not being alone (see page 348). Or you could go to a group or 1 to 1 therapist to get some honesty around your relationship with it.

Let's talk about sex

This is a complex area and hugely personal to each of us, but I don't believe it's talked about enough once you reach a certain age. And yet our sexuality is a significant part of who we are.

There will probably be times in all of our lives when we feel less interested in having sex than others. And times when we feel less sexual. If your relationship has recently ended and you weren't having sex very regularly (as so often happens when a relationship comes to an end) you can subconsciously shut down this part of yourself. If sex with someone else is really not something you want to do any more that's absolutely fine; the key is not to deny a part of who we are because it feels safer, or we lack confidence.

Sex drive is very connected to your hormone levels. You might be wanting a lot of sex and your partner isn't, and if your partner is a man he might need to get his testosterone levels checked. And if you have lost your sex drive, it's worth checking your hormone levels are right. There are so many women I speak to at 50+ who go on HRT, their sex drive returns and they feel like they are having an affair as the sex is so satisfying. It can come back ...

Whatever feeling sexual means to you – whether it's something you want to do on your own or with someone else – that is a great thing to explore. Shutting down this side of us blocks our energy.

All I can say to you is that when I am not feeling sexual energy, I feel I am ageing quicker. You need to be in tune with your sexuality. It does not mean having an affair, it just means feeling confident in your body. If you watch something that you used to find sexy and no longer do, you have shut off an element of your body and you need to find it again. Wake up that good friend.

You need to be in tune with your sexuality

Feeling all the rage

Our hormones make their presence most felt when there is a significant change in the levels in our bodies. So when we go through puberty, are pregnant, are perimenopausal or menopausal. And some of us experience breakouts, mood swings, inflammation and a whole host more at various points in our monthly cycle.

But whether we are aware of it or not, hormones affect everything we do and balanced hormone levels are important for our overall wellbeing. They have an impact on so many things beyond fertility and mood.

I started going through the perimenopause when I was 45. I know that some women who experience the low moods and lack of energy often associated with perimenopause and menopause are initially misdiagnosed by their doctor and put on antidepressants, which does nothing to get to the root of the problem. Knowledge of the subject varies from doctor to doctor. Which is why it's so important to educate yourself and be proactive about getting help when you need it.

It's a huge topic and I am not an expert, but it is important that we talk about this more so I asked Dr Erika Schwartz if she would give us her thoughts (she has written three amazing books on the subject of hormones if you want to delve deeper). I first went to see Dr Erika in New York after I found I was getting nowhere with getting on the right HRT for me and it made a huge difference. As women, we don't have to simply accept terrible PMT or low sex drive or lack of energy or mental fog or any of the other things caused by a hormone imbalance – there are solutions.

What we need to know about hormones by Dr Erika Schwartz

We are our hormones.

When our hormones are in balance we are young, healthy, full of energy, sleep well, don't have wrinkles, can party all night, go to work in the morning and we generally love sex. When our hormones are out of balance or they leave us, we start having symptoms like hot flashes, night sweats, insomnia, irritability, depression, anxiety, weight gain, crazy allergies, itching, general malaise and more. We may believe this means we are just getting old and it goes with the territory. But we don't have to suffer and we don't have to go into our twilight years sick, bent over with crumbling bones and losing our minds. There are plenty of solutions and great ways to get old feeling healthy and energetic.

For starters, let's eliminate fear from the equation. There was a study in 2002 which was retracted in 2013 that scared doctors and women as it implied that hormone replacement therapy was linked to cancer. But we now know it was all wrong. What are known as bioidentical, human identical or natural hormones are believed to help prevent cancer, heart disease, osteoporosis, Alzheimer's, and they decrease all-cause mortality in women who start taking them before menopause (NICE, 2015). I've been working with them for almost 30 years, have been taking them myself for 26 years and have treated more than 10,000 women with them.

When we are talking about ageing, it's not just about the hormones. They open the door to turning back the clock; the rest is diet, exercise, supplements, peptides, sleep and stress management.

Oestradiol (the most powerful of the three types of oestrogen), progesterone and testosterone are the key hormones to know about, though there are others too.

Our twenties

Irregular periods are not a sign something is wrong and don't necessarily indicate a hormone imbalance. This is the time to learn to live inside your body, to focus on lifestyle, to learn about your body and how diet, exercise, sleep, stress affect it. Bear in mind that if you start taking birth control or use a contraceptive implant that relies on hormones, this is suppressing your body's normal hormone production.

Our thirties

Our hormone levels and ovulation start to change. If you are trying to have a baby you can get a blood test to find out your FSH, LH and prolactin levels toward the end of your cycle or day two of your period. Some women experience worse PMS symptoms – irritability, short temper, weight gain, sleep issues, occasional hot flashes, night sweats – the cause of which is hormonal and can be corrected with hormones. Swapping hormonal birth control for a copper coil is worth considering as this is least likely to alter your hormone levels.

If you have a baby and struggle to recover your pre-pregnancy body and mind, find a doctor or practitioner who knows about hormone balance. This is much better than just thinking this is the way life is.

Our forties

Changes we began to experience in our thirties now become more noticeable. Forget about regular cycles and focus on how you feel, with particular attention to diet. Take supplements and adjust your diet to give you all the nutrients possible. Hormones are made in the gut, and the gut biome, the healthy bacteria, has an impact. You may notice insulin resistance, which manifests in the spare tyre around your middle. This is often caused by carbs - namely bread, pasta, alcohol, dairy. Processed foods are more difficult to tolerate.

Our fifties

Most women go into menopause around 50. But I have seen many women in their forties who have already stopped having a period and women in their late fifties who still have regular periods. So let's forget the labels and just focus on keeping healthy, vibrant and full of energy regardless of our hormone status or menstrual frequency. Besides going on the correct regimen of bioidentical hormones for you, you now need thyroid and adrenal hormones and to focus on lifestyle to keep you healthy and protected from illnesses associated with old age.

Our sixties, seventies and onwards

If you have built good habits and understand the connection between everything you do and how you feel, the crucial role of hormones and the importance of finding your own sweet spot in life, you can adjust as your body's requirements change. Keep taking those hormones and supplements, and do everything you need to keep you enjoying the marvellous life you created for yourself. Illnesses like diabetes, osteoporosis and heart disease are not an inevitable part of growing older - remember that we can play an active part in defending ourselves against them.

The supplements worth taking

I take a number of vitamin and mineral supplements to support my body (some have suggested that I rattle). People often ask whether you can get everything you need from a good diet but I just don't think you necessarily do. For one reason, by the time fresh food gets to me, living as I do in a city, it's already typically three to five days old. And then it might sit in the fridge for a couple of days. In this time, a lot of the nutrients have gone. Our bodies have complex needs - which scientists are still learning more about all the time - and supplements allow us to fill any gaps not met by our nutritional intake.

Also, if we want to help our bodies remain fit and healthy as we go down the path of life, taking the right supplements is one way we can support it.

There are many, many different products out there and deciding which - if any - are right for you will take some research. I have learned a lot through working with Shabir Daya, a pharmacist and the co-founder of Victoria Health, a brilliant place for advice and a provider of natural health products in the UK. I asked him to give a brief introduction to some of the key supplements and explain why you might decide to take them.

Our bodies have complex needs

What supplements to take by Shabir Daya

I am a firm believer that there are some fundamental nutrients and supplements that most of us would benefit from taking daily. They include a vitamin D3 supplement, an omega 3 supplement and, for a lot of us, a quality probiotic.

Vitamin D3 was thought to be required for strong bones and teeth but now we know that virtually every gland in our body has a vitamin D receptor, meaning that it is used in a wide range of processes. Numerous studies indicate that many of us do not get sufficient vitamin D from our diet. Whilst the World Health Organization recommends 600iu of vitamin D3 at every age, most scientists in the field believe that a woman of average height and weight can take 2000iu per day.

Omega 3 is required by the body for the manufacture of hormones, for transporting oily soluble vitamins in and out of cells, for maintaining healthy skin, for improving circulation and for lowering inflammation levels. It is found in oily fish like tuna, mackerel and salmon, but most of us don't eat these two or three times a week, so a supplement is useful.

Probiotics are beneficial bacteria involved in some very crucial processes, such as maintaining a healthy immune system, detoxification in the gut, promoting healthy bowel movement, providing energising B vitamins and a lot more. Lots of scientific research is currently happening in this area; we are finding specific strains of bacteria influence mood, cholesterol and even gum health.

Eating a **balanced, healthy diet** is very important at every age. As we get older, we can consider adding more supplements to support the body's natural processes.

A calcium supplement is a good thing to introduce when you reach your forties if you have a family history of osteoporosis or are on a dairy-free diet.

Vitamin C is great for the function of blood vessels, skin, teeth and bones, and is thought to help protect cells from oxidative stress.

NAD+ is found in virtually all living cells and is important to sustaining life. Falling NAD+ levels have been linked with age-related diseases and it is this property that may help to prevent accelerated ageing. Levels of NAD+ have halved by our 40's so it is worth introducing supplements such as nicotinamide riboside.

Our digestive system produces lower amounts of digestive enzymes as we age. If you suffer from bloating and other digestive concerns, **a quality digestive enzymes supplement** suitable for daily use will not only help to prevent this, but can enhance absorption of vitamins and minerals.

A protein called **intrinsic factor** takes **vitamin B12** from the intestines into the bloodstream. Vitamin B12 works to enhance red blood cells which carry oxygen to all parts of the body; it helps in the manufacture of hormones for energy and stress reduction; it protects the nervous system and is required for the manufacture of the sleep hormone. When you reach your fifties, the production of intrinsic factor slows so you may wish to ask your GP or health practitioner for a vitamin B12 test. If you are deficient, there is no point in taking tablets as these will not be absorbed efficiently. Opt for vitamin B12 sprays or lozenges as the vitamin can get absorbed from under the tongue or the sides of cheeks directly into the bloodstream.

Supplements can also be used to address specific concerns. Here are some of the most common I recommend people try.

Bad skin often comes down to hormonal disturbances, causing the release of inflammatory chemicals that lead to excess sebum production, clogging pores. Zinc is a mineral which is known to calm inflamed skin when applied topically (think zinc and castor oil cream for an inflamed baby's bottom) or you can take a supplement which contains zinc.

Premenstrual syndrome is a collection of emotional and physical concerns associated with a hormonal imbalance, specifically when the body has more oestrogen than progesterone. Three nutrients thought to help alleviate the symptoms are magnesium, vitamin B6 and saffron. Magnesium relaxes muscles and nerves while helping to alleviate cramping and breast tenderness; vitamin B6 is thought to regulate the sex hormones and saffron elevates mood.

Iron deficiency anaemia results in a lack of sufficient red blood cells to carry oxygen around the body, leading to shortness of breath and a lack of energy. The most common causes are heavy periods and pregnancy. I recommend ionic iron, a non-constipating iron supplement which provides iron in the most bioavailable state.

Bloating is most commonly caused by a lack of digestive enzymes, which can occur because of stress, hormonal disturbances or simply the ageing process. A quality digestive enzymes supplement will help to alleviate bloating and also enhance nutrient uptake, usually by hundreds of per cent.

The exact cause of **rosacea** is still not fully understood. Genetics, intestinal bacterial overgrowth, skin mites and irregularities between the nervous system and the blood vessels are all possible culprits. Supplements containing zinc and herbs such as burdock are often found to improve this concern.

Mental fog is a very common concern when under stress, at times of sleep disturbances or during phases of hormonal changes. People feel they cannot focus on a task; they may be forgetful or feel less mentally sharp. I recommend a supplement called lion's mane - a mushroom extract available in powder form for tea - to enhance focus, clarity of thought and mental energy.

As a rule of thumb, take supplements with food - especially herbal supplements since they are foreign to the body and can cause gastric disturbances. Only amino acids such as glutamine and lysine should be taken on an empty stomach, ideally about half an hour before any food. Though many vitamins are available in sublingual forms (as a drop or lozenge placed under the tongue) only a handful of vitamins are absorbed through this method. Try to spread out supplements - taking them all at once is inefficient as the digestive system can only cope with a certain amount.

If you are taking medications and you have checked it is still fine to take supplements, take them at least two hours from the time at which you take your medications, in case they affect absorption.

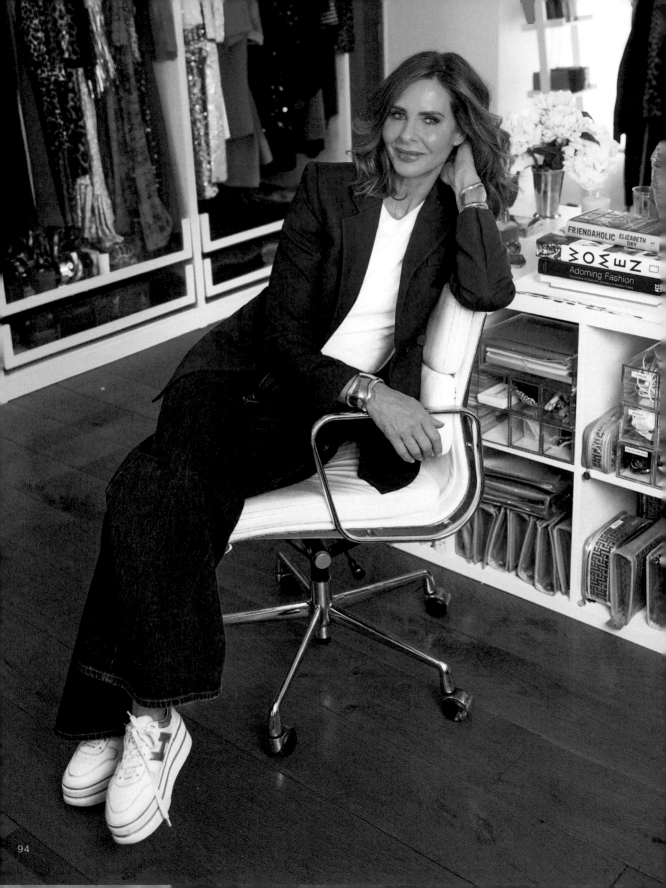

Bills, bills, bills

How comfortable are you talking about money?

Are you someone who is on top of their finances or do you avoid opening that online banking app until you really have to?

If you shuddered slightly when you read that heading you are hardly alone. Money is such an emotive topic and a source of fear for many of us – and not just the very understandable worry that we might not have enough of it to pay the bills.

Your parents' relationship with money and whether you grew up feeling there was enough of it or you picked up that things were very stretched does of course have a big impact on your attitude towards spending and saving as an adult.

My family were comfortable when I was young. I had a nanny and then I went to boarding school from an early age. I didn't see my parents much but I definitely grew up with financial privilege. Then, when I was about 18, a few business deals of my father's didn't go so well and money became tight. We weren't completely broke but I remember feeling out of balance and it was a very difficult time of readjustment for me.

Although I was never good at school, I have always been a grafter. When I was 16 I did a Saturday job at Partridges, a high-end grocery store in central London. This made me quite unusual among my school friends, none of whom had jobs. I wanted to earn my own money.

Even when I didn't need to worry about money so much, as I was working a lot and earning a good salary in my thirties, I always had this underlying feeling of anxiety. Future financial uncertainty stops you from enjoying and accepting the present. Instead I was always worrying. And then in my forties I separated from my husband and my TV work dried up in the UK. I felt a real financial insecurity as I tried to figure out what I would do next.

I felt relief when Susannah and I were offered contracts to make our show around the world. I became the main breadwinner. The downside of this was that for about seven months of the year, I spent Monday to Friday working abroad and then the weekend at home with Lyla. It was a really difficult decision for me to make at the time, but there was no alternative.

I have definitely made good and bad financial decisions over the years. I have spent money both frivolously and wisely. I have spent a lot of money on clothes, of course, although many I sold when I was raising money to start Trinny London.

I don't think talking about money should be taboo. And I don't think we should let it intimidate us. Like any fear, worries about finances grow more powerful when they are allowed to fester in the dark. Anxiety around money can be crippling and cast a shadow over so many areas of our life, sapping our energy. Even making financial decisions when you do have money can feel fraught and stressful.

The key is not to get overwhelmed and to try to separate the emotion from the problem or decision as much as you can, to allow you to see it more clearly. As far as possible, take a calm, logical approach, as you would to any other situation that didn't involve your bank balance.

There was a time in my life when I went to Debtors Anonymous (DA). It is a very good self-help group that will help you to put your finances in perspective and understand your relationship with money. When we feel concerned about money, we're not so capable because we live in a place of fear. You need to get an objective view.

Take a calm and logical approach

ASK YOURSELF

1 Do you know exactly where your money goes every month?

2 Do you always feel guilty spending money, even if it is an essential purchase?

3 Do you hide non-essential purchases from your partner, or yourself, by putting clothes in the back of your wardrobe?

4 Do you always struggle to juggle your bills?

CHALLENGE YOURSELF

Focus

Spend one week just focusing on your finances. It's only a week in your life and it's really going to help you. Write down everything – the monthly standing orders you have to pay and then look at your salary to see what is left over to spend on non-essentials. If you find there's nothing, ask yourself if you are challenging yourself enough on your work value. If you think you're doing a really good job and you're underpaid, consider listing all the brilliant things you're good at and when you have a review, sell yourself to get a good raise. And if they can't pay you, it is time to consider changing job.

Make a decision for now

Every day for a month write down everything that you spend. Do this in the notes on your phone. We often forget the little things and they add up. It could be the third coffee of the day or going out for dinner twice in one week. What are you spending money on? You might spend money on clothing, but you want to go on holiday. Think about how your spending brings you happiness.

Keeping up with technology

New apps, devices, platforms - even jargon and ideas - arrive with such speed and regularity that you don't even have to be far down the path of life to start to feel overwhelmed or out of date. But it is vital not to throw your hands in the air and give up.

I see this with friends who are my age and older (and younger!) all too often. We feel challenged by some new technology and are afraid of looking stupid.

Technology is a part of every element of our life. You might be of an age where if you're trying to do something on your phone, your teenager will lean in and do it because you are being too slow. We can get used to this, but this will make you feel even less connected. I think it's critical to have an understanding of what's going on around me. If you think that you just about get Facebook, Instagram and TikTok, but that ChatGPT, AI and the Metaverse is something beyond you, just think that in five years these will be just as familiar as Instagram is to you now. So learn about them and feel involved. Have an opinion. The world is moving forward.

Keeping up with technology is not the opposite of having a spiritual life - the two can run in parallel. I do think people can get addicted to social media. It isn't always true to reality and we should be cautious of those who present an unrealistic version of life or opinions that aren't based on truth, but really this is not about that. This is about feeling that you are capable, that you can do it yourself and that you are in control.

Technology is part of every element of our life

I'll be there for you

Friendship is so important. That feeling of community, of having people in your life who know you and reflect back to you who you really are is invaluable.

I have not always been good at reaching out to a friend when I have felt isolated, low or stressed. It can become a vicious circle, but we really must reach out. I make a conscious effort to put energy into my friendships and I have learnt the power of being candid.

Women who are single often build up stronger female friendship groups. Having a partner who you live with can make you complacent. Friendships do take work to sustain. But it is the most fulfilling kind of work when you create relationships that will be with you through every stage. Just keep the communication lines open.

We can feel awkward about reaching out to an old friend who we haven't seen for a while. But I absolutely think we should and if they don't respond then that's fine – you tried. You might be the type of friend who is always there for other people, and you never ask for help. Ask yourself why wouldn't your friends want to help you? Remember that people need to feel needed and it helps their self-worth. Sharing is a generous, not selfish, act for both of you.

You should have friendships with people who are much older and younger than you. Age should not be a barrier to making a connection and nor should life experiences. You do not need to connect on every level to be able to create a meaningful friendship. However, it is important to go to the right person to get your needs met. Your practical friend may be great at offering help in a crisis, but might not be the right person to call when you need someone to listen to how you feel rather than to try to 'solve' it.

It's important to show enough of yourself to let the people you want in your life see and understand you. This can feel difficult if you are someone who feels shy. The only way people can think 'that's my kind of woman' is if they see a bit of vulnerability. I'm not suggesting we should be oversharing with every acquaintance but we are all drawn to those who can show emotional confidence.

The friendship wheel

It is important to evaluate friendships and their balance at different periods. You need to take care of yourself and decide what percentage each friendship should take up in your life.

The friendship wheel will highlight a few things to you. One, do you have too many friends that drain you? If so, how can you let them go? This can be one of the hardest things to do as it requires a mixture of honesty and kindness. If there is a friend who's a bit toxic and drains all your energy, you do need to remove them from your life. I have written letters to those people in my life and I have explained honestly: 'I feel right now that you need to be with people who can give you something that I don't feel equipped to do.'

Two, are you feeling a little bit lonely? This can be very difficult to admit. But this is fundamentally different from feeling alone. Loneliness can be helped by many things. A big element is asking yourself, are you doing enough to really love yourself? The other element is thinking you would like some more friends in your life. How will you go about that? There are many gentle places to start to develop friendships. I will mention the Trinny Tribe group on Facebook, which is a community who have come together over the common belief that it's a safe place for them to be the women they want to be today, and not the women that their partners, children, mothers, siblings or friends expect them to be. We can feel lonely, not like ourselves or even the person that we want to be with those who are already in our lives. There can be too much obligation from the history that you share. Take a look around and see this as a chance to test out the person that you've always secretly wanted to be.

Use the chart to help take action. If you were to draw arrows along the line, would the energy be travelling in just one direction, or two? Any arrows that point solely away from you mean the relationship is no longer giving you what you need. We should also use this to question what we are contributing to the relationship.

Friends from school and uni. They have strong opinions about themselves and you.

Friends who know how to have a great time.

Friends from childhood. There are many memories, but your lives are now different.

Friends who are older than you.

Friends that listen and give you time.

Friends that never help themselves and never learn.

Friends that you can see anywhere, anytime, without effort.

Me

Friends that you meet at the school gate. Vital at one time, but are they still now?

Friends who are slow to respond and you always make the effort.

Friends who are permanently surrounded by drama.

Friends from family obligation, where you keep in touch even though there is no common ground.

Friends who make you smile whenever you see their number.

Friends who are younger than you.

Friends who are overtly lovely, but always seem to critique you and often say 'you should'.

FEAR
LESS

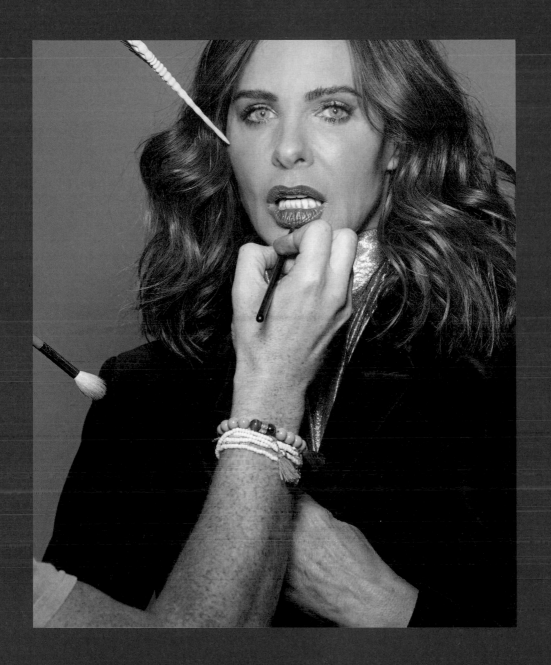

BEAUTY

GOOD SKINCARE IS FUNDAMENTAL

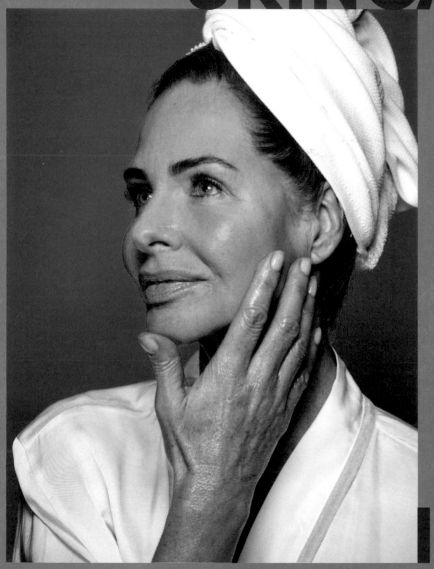

Skincare

When we look after our skin we are nurturing ourselves.

We all want to look in the mirror and see the best version of the woman we can be. If we see a tired, dull complexion then that is how we will feel. When you bring out the life and glow in our face, everything else will follow.

Yes, there are some things that no product can help you with – for example, nothing that comes in a jar or a tube will fix deep frown lines. But, crucially, no amount of tweakments will give you fresh, healthy-looking skin if you are not cleansing, exfoliating and moisturising consistently and correctly. Nor will the best makeup in the world hide skin that isn't cared for.

Your skin will go through changes as you age and you have to adapt to what your skin is dealing with at that time. From the age of 13 to 30 I had chronic cystic acne that could only be improved by Roaccutane (a prescription drug), and from that point on I never took my skin for granted. In my early forties, I had to adapt as I experienced hyperpigmentation in pregnancy, and then again in my mid forties when the acne returned during the early stages of my menopause.

A good skincare routine is a positive, affirming activity. I want to demystify skincare and give you easy-to-understand morning and evening routines, so that you can transform how you look and feel better about your skin, and consequently, yourself.

Use products that are customised to your needs, not your friends

FEEL INSPIRED

In this part, I want you to think about how your skin feels to you right now.

It's best to focus on one or two skincare goals at a time rather than trying to do it all at once. You will avoid overloading your skin and you'll be able to see when your new routine is providing results.

Our skin is a reflection of how we feel and our unique life experience. It can show our toughest moments as well as our greatest joys.

Ongoing stresses of everyday life, work, family, lack of sleep, and poor diet can change the way our skin genes work. These stress factors have the ability to switch on the genes that can worsen our skin concerns, increase inflammation and accelerate ageing.

We can't always control what's happening in our lives, but we can reset the impact stress has on our skin. Choosing the right ingredients to go into your skincare products can have a hugely transformative effect on your skin, while actually improving the long-term quality of your skin.

I have interviewed hundreds of skincare experts, tried thousands of skincare products and spoken to thousands of women over the last twenty-five years. I have learnt that it's so important to listen to your skin, as you go down the path of life you need to be informed and take action.

Decoding skincare

Trends come and go in skincare, just like in fashion. The big beauty brands have huge marketing budgets to spend on pushing their products (something that, as a founder of a startup beauty brand, I know only too well!). There are so many products to choose from.

This is why I think educating yourself on the key active ingredients that go into skincare is absolutely worth your time. It is imperative to do and this knowledge will help you make good decisions and avoid wasting money on something that looks fancy and smells delightful, but has little going for it.

The key question to always consider is what do you want from the products you apply to your skin? Perhaps your main bugbear is dry skin. Or you feel your complexion is dull. Maybe you have milia or acne. Make a plan to target your specific concerns.

Knowing what active ingredients are is key here. Your skincare routine should be made up of a small number of good quality products that work together to give you the results you wish to see, with nothing that you don't need. It's important to avoid overloading your skin or stripping away the natural oils altogether.

There is a lot of complex science behind skincare. Since I started learning about skincare in my 20's, formulations have come a long way. The crucial thing is not the brand you buy from. The key thing to consider is what is in the formulations and how those ingredients work together.

It is all about the ingredients

The essentials

Here is the overview of the elements that I believe are essential for great skin. You can find more details about all of the products and the breakdown of possible ingredients at the end of this section (see pages 138–151).

1   A cleanser

I recommend a balm cleanser to help melt away the makeup and dirt from your skin. You can invest in a few to cover specific concerns, or use the same one. In the evening you must always cleanse your skin twice.

2   An exfoliating acid

These come in the form of AHAs, BHAs and PHAs. They aide in removing the dead skin cells that make your skin look dull and feel dry.

3   Vitamin C serum

This is an essential part of any good morning routine.

4   A retinoid serum

This is an essential part of any good evening routine.

5   Moisturiser

Find a weight of moisturiser for your skin type (see page 16).

6   SPF 30 or 50

No matter the weather or your age, you must wear an SPF of at least 30, but ideally 50, everyday. This will make a huge difference to how your skin will age, as a good proportion of skin ageing is down to sun damage.

It is time to face facts

Big hormonal changes – puberty, pregnancy, menopause will show on our skin – but there will be subtle shifts too. Our priorities and skincare goals will alter as we notice ourselves moving into a new phase. It is important to address lifestyle issues like stress at the same time, as this can make a big difference to our skin. Two months is the rough time frame before you can expect to see real results – just be patient with the right active ingredients.

Twenties

I do hope you arrive into your twenties no longer feeling that your skin is so much at the mercy of your hormones – as someone who was still dealing with acne into my early thirties, if you are not there yet work out what skin type you have (see page 16). The steps to then follow are:

1   Gentle cleansing.

2   Use an exfoliant 2-3 times a week.

3   Find a good moisturiser that suits your skin type.

4   Wear the highest SPF you can – at least 30, but ideally 50.

Thirties

You may start to notice the levels of elastin and collagen begin to drop off – from our mid-twenties we lose 1% of collagen every year. This is the decade to start using vitamin C in the morning and a mild retinoid at night. The vitamin C will help prevent and reduce the sun damage that is going to start to show as you go down the path of life. Using a mild retinoid serum at night is also a good strategy. You may also have had a baby and have had to address issues like hyperpigmentation or acne brought on by pregnancy. The key is not to rush off for the latest tweakment you've seen on Instagram or TikTok at the sight of your first wrinkle.

Forties

Many of us find that we no longer bounce back in the same way we once did from a few late nights, a boozy evening or a period of poor diet. They can show on our face in the form of deeper lines, dehydration, puffiness and our skin starts to lose its elasticity. This is when we look to up the ante in terms of active ingredients in our skincare. You might want to introduce some peptides or hyaluronic acid to help boost the skin elasticity, or stronger vitamin C or stronger retinoids could be introduced. Lifestyle factors become increasingly important too. It sounds simple but do make sure you are drinking enough water, eating a vitamin-rich diet and getting enough sleep whenever you can. It's time to start paying more attention to your neck too. And do not forget the SPF.

Fifties

Most of us will notice our skin becoming thinner and slightly drier. Those strong active ingredients it tolerated without complaint in our thirties and forties may start to feel too harsh. The core routine should now be: vitamin C in the AM to encourage collagen production and retinoid in the PM. Replenish the skin in the evening with a nourishing moisturiser that contains ceramides and/or peptides. Embrace the oxygenating, blood-flow enhancing benefits of facial massage and don't forget the hands. Some of us sail through the menopause, for others it comes as a shock to the system. If you need to overhaul your skincare routine as a result, introduce changes slowly. Once you go into menopause, it increases to 2% loss per year for collagen. Imagine the cushion losing a bit of it's feathers every year. And do not forget the SPF.

Lifestyle issues make a difference to our skin

Sixties

By now you will have lost 50% of your collagen, so you will likely be noticing a reduction in structure and firmness. Paying attention to lifestyle as well as skincare is important for maintaining our glow. Practise facial exercise to add tone from within. Dehydrated skin looks more lined, so hydrate inside and out by drinking plenty of water and make your moisturiser work harder by finding one that contains skin nourishing ceramides, hyaluronic acid and peptides. Lack of oestrogen can lead to insomnia, so make sure you have a good sleep routine. Feeling and looking tired are the enemy, so concentrate on the things that make you and your skin look and feel energised. And do not forget the SPF.

Seventies and beyond

It's important to respect and be kind to our skin at every age, but particularly so at this stage in our lives. Use gentle motions when cleansing, massaging or applying creams and serums to the skin, especially around the eye area. Balms and rich lotions will feel luxurious rather than cloying. Ceramides, lightweight squalene oil and hyaluronic acid will rehydrate and repair. Nurture your skin and protect it from the elements - do not forget the SPF.

The average skin cycle is 28 days – in your twenties it's 21 days and 45 days in your fifties – it takes 3 skin cycles to see results

ASK YOURSELF

1   Do you know your skin type (see page 16)?

2   What are your biggest skin concerns?

3   Do you know what ingredients to look out for to help you address your skin goals?

4   Do you have a consistent AM and PM skincare routine?

CHALLENGE YOURSELF

1   If you only manage to cleanse and moisturise but that's about it, start improving your routine by first using a gentle exfoliator 2–3 times a week.

2   Applying vitamin C every morning is one of the best things you can do for your skin. There are great products available across all budgets, so challenge yourself to find one that suits you.

3   If you have been using the same products for ages and you are not sure they are the right thing for your skin anymore, look at what is and is not working.

4   If you are overdoing it with a nightly routine involving around seven or eight different products, then follow my suggested routine on page 116 instead.

Your morning routine

I am asked a lot about what a skincare routine should consist of. So here is a basic routine to get you started. Think about what ingredients might help you, so you can personalise this routine to your skin.

In terms of what order you use your products, in the AM or PM, the general rule is that if you're layering, work from lightest to heaviest in terms of texture. The lightest products should go on first, allowing the products following to be absorbed.

Some of you will just put your head under the shower every morning. Whereas some of you will do a ritualistic morning wake up routine. Most of you will sit somewhere in the middle. Every morning, I would beg you to include the following steps. Clean and prep your skin properly. Overnight, your skin releases toxins and they sit on the top of the skin, sometimes seen as a slightly filmy texture. There's oil in this, so water won't remove it. This routine will create a perfect surface so that your skincare will penetrate properly. Good cleansing goes a long way.

The rest of this morning routine depends on what elements you are thinking of addressing, but it must always end with an SPF of at least 30, ideally 50. 90% of our skin ageing is caused by sunlight, so always apply this.

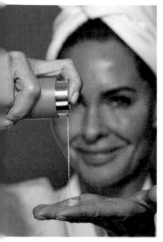

Stage 1: **Cleanse**

A single cleanse is enough as your skin hasn't been exposed to all the nasty things that will be thrown its way in the course of a day. If your skin is normal to dry, I would suggest a balm cleanser which you can massage into your skin and take off with a hot cloth. If you're normal to oily, go for a gel cleanser with a gentle acid.

Stage 2: **PHA Exfoliate**

This is not a step for everyone, but you can use a PHA in the morning. This is far more effective than using a toner here.

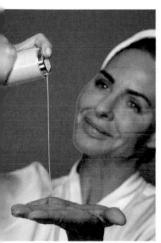

Stage 3: **Vitamin C Serum**

A vitamin C serum in the morning is what the skin needs to help fight the damage that is inflicted during the day.

Stage 4: **Moisturiser**

Many people think moisturiser is the most important element of their routine. Find a moisturiser that suits your skin type. Moisturisers will help protect your skin barrier and keep your skin feeling hydrated and moisturised. Moisturisers are very personal, so chose one that absorbs well so that your skin doesn't feel dry.

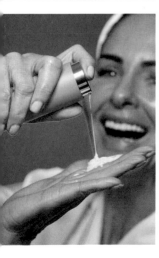

Stage 5: **SPF 30 or 50**

SPF has come a long way, there are so many great formulations that are SPF 30 or 50 and still feel weightless. Make sure you choose an SPF that it is broad spectrum with UVA (ageing) and UVB (burning) protection and ideally with blue light protection (from screen damage). You need to use a bigger amount than your moisturiser for the SPF to work. It's the equivalent of ¼ of a teaspoon for your face, and ½ a teaspoon for your face and neck.

Your evening routine

Your evening routine will consist of more steps as most of us have more time in the evening. However, try not to think of your skincare routine as a chore, something standing between you and finally being able to get into bed at the end of a long day. This is an opportunity to take a few minutes just for yourself. Take the time to massage your face, let go of the stresses of the day and prepare your mind for sleep.

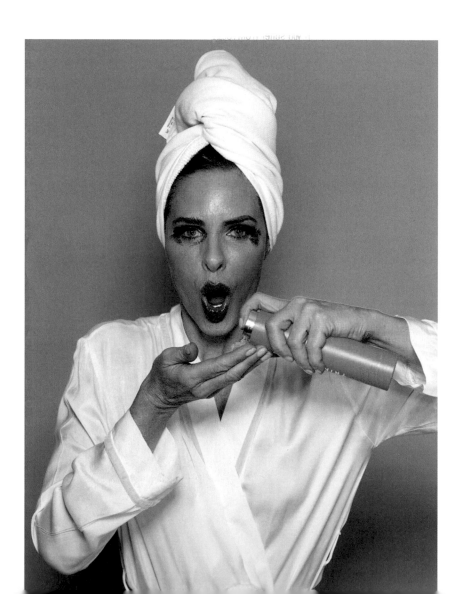

Stage 1: **Double cleanse**

Balm cleansers are oil based and oil attracts oil, so begin with a balm cleanser to melt away the day's make up and grime. Wipe away with a face or washcloth and warm water and follow up with a gel cleanser to get rid of any residual cleanser and get into the pores. Cleaning our skin in a thorough but kind way is the cornerstone of a good skincare routine. I promise the double cleanse takes so little effort and is absolutely worth it. You can use the same product twice, if you prefer. This might sound obvious, but do not to wash your face in water that is too hot. You will stress your skin and likely dry it out. If you suffer from rosacea be particularly mindful of this.

Stage 2: **Exfoliate for skin type**

Exfoliation used to mean using a granular exfoliant, which only dealt with the very top layer of the skin. But here I'm talking about liquid exfoliant that stays on and it should be based on what is best for your skin type (see page 16). This will clear out any dead skin cells and is essential for brightening your complexion. It also preps your skin for the products to follow.

Stage 3: **Serum for skin concern**

Now look at retinoids and how you can add them to your routine. Select one that is specific to your skin issues (see page 124).

Stage 4: **Moisturiser (optional)**

I don't use a really heavy cream or facial oil at night because I think our skin needs to have time to breathe. But if you feel your skin needs it, add this step. I recommend a much lighter formula that can easily penetrate, as you should be careful of the weight you put on top of your skin. Overnight is the best opportunity for our skin to rid itself of any toxins and regenerate.

False friends

Here are a few beauty products that I do not think are worth your time.

Micellar water: If you are somewhere you can't properly cleanse, micellar water will get off some of that top level of makeup, but all of the rest of the day's toxins and SPF are still sitting there on your skin. Sure, you can see lots of makeup on the cotton pad, but it's not giving you anywhere near the deep cleanse you need.

Facial wipes: Another 'in emergencies only' product. Not only will facial wipes smear a lot of the dirt across your face, removing only a small amount of it, they are bad for the environment too.

Collagen creams: Collagen molecules are very large. They will not make it through your skin's barrier cells. We can use peptides and vitamin C to support the production of collagen and we can take collagen in the form of supplements. But a cream or serum is not going to be effective.

Pore strips: I know, the idea of clearing out your pores in one fell swoop is enticing. But this is where short-term satisfaction comes at the expense of long-term results. Most peel-off pore masks and extraction tools are gimmicks and, at worst, can cause damage. Anything that encourages you to prod, rip or tear at your skin is bad news, leading to things like inflammation, redness and even broken blood vessels. To avoid damage, it is much better to get a professional to carry out extractions every few months.

The added extras

I love a tool. They add something extra to a skincare routine. I use many different ones and some weeks I will use something every day and other times I will go weeks without. Whenever I do use them consistently, I notice I can get my skin to the next level - sitting between a skincare routine and an in-clinic treatment.

The majority of the time a tool is a bigger investment. If you are somebody who even struggles with the basic skincare routine, this is not for you yet. Don't invest if you won't use it, try this first:

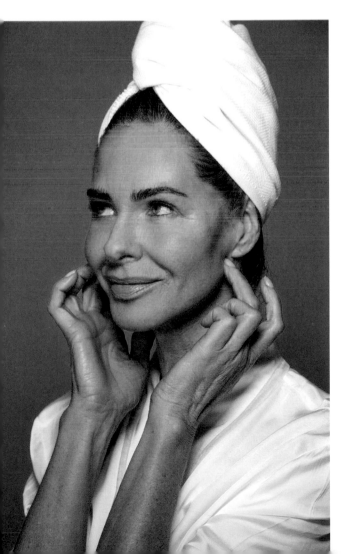

Finger facial massage

I'm going to start with the one that's free. All of you can do this. Facial massage really works but only if you commit to doing it.

This will get your lymph system working and is for somebody who suffers from what I call 'wake up puff'. It might be that you sleep very flat or you eat inflammatory foods at night. The first thing you need to do is get the lymphatic system working. This is brilliant for oxygenating your skin. You will see redness, but it will quickly go.

Step 1: The lymph nodes are around your earlobes. Make tiny circular motions around the front and around the back of your earlobes. Do this very gently for 2 minutes.

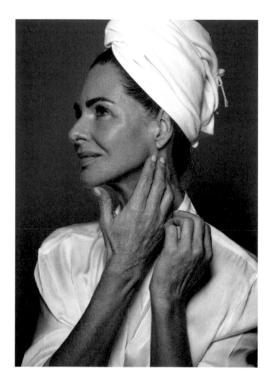

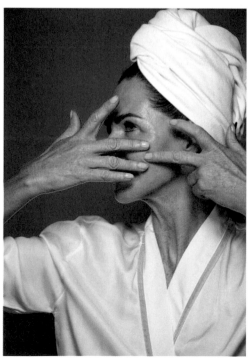

Step 2: Start on one side first and always keep your fingers in contact with your skin. Gently move three of your fingers up to your front of your earlobe and down your neck all the way to your clavicle (collarbone) and repeat that process. Keep a rhythm and do this 20 times. This will move the toxins that are contributing to your puffiness. Your face will now feel awake.

Step 3: You can now move onto the eye area, but you must complete step 2 to see the benefit. If your lymph is blocked, the puffiness under your eyes has nowhere to go. This step is much quicker. Go to the inner corner of your eye, and press your two middle fingers gently on the outside of your nose. Slightly lift, but not off the skin, and move slowly underneath the eye and press again. Repeat until you reach the outer corner.

Step 4: You're now going to take your middle finger of one hand and your ring finger and your middle finger on the other hand, and you create a scissoring motion to cause friction. Start on your forehead. You shouldn't actually be dragging your skin because you're continuously lightly pulling in opposite directions. Just go up and down and to the left and to the right for about a minute.

Step 5: Massage any other areas, such as your cheeks, to finish.

Vocal facial massage

This next part of the routine will work the different muscles in your face and neck, and improve the elasticity and structure of your skin. If you do this properly, the next day you will feel the satisfying ache in your face like you would normally get in your limbs after going to the gym.

Here you are going to say (loudly project) the vowels of the alphabet, AEIOU. I take it further than my grandmother taught me, and will do 10 A's, 10 E's, 10 I's, 10 O's and finally 10 U's. You are going to really exaggerate how you form each letter, so that each of them will impact different muscles on your face and neck.

The A: This works on your neck. When you make the A sound, push your tongue towards the back of your throat and the two long muscles of your neck will come to life. These are the muscles that get ignored as we age.

The E: This will work the muscle in your jaw. Push back your mouth as you make the sound. You want to stretch the muscles in a mixture of shortening and lengthening movements.

The I: This should come from your belly and almost feel like you're in pain. You want your partner to hear you shouting and wonder if you are having an argument!

The O: This is not from your chest, but from your stomach. Pull in your stomach as you make this sound.

The U: Pull in your pelvic floor muscles as you make the sound. You almost want it to feel like you are protecting your muscles by pulling them in.

Do each of these 10 times. I would suggest you do them in the privacy of your own home, although I have been known to do it on aeroplanes. It really is an unbelievable release. I wish I remembered to do it every day.

Gua shua

If you don't want to use your hands for the lymphatic facial massage, try gua sha. This is based on an ancient Chinese healing technique whereby blood flow and lymphatic drainage are stimulated by using a curved tool made from stones like jade, rose quartz or amethyst. You should apply gentle pressure when using this tool, and use both short and long strokes. Like with finger facial massage, you will want to get your lymphatic system working in the first instance. Apply a serum or facial oil and then use the tool on your face and neck. Ideally, use this daily or two or three times a week. Spend just five minutes doing this routine and you will be sure to see the difference. Be sure to be gentle and keep in mind that you may look slightly flushed just after using.

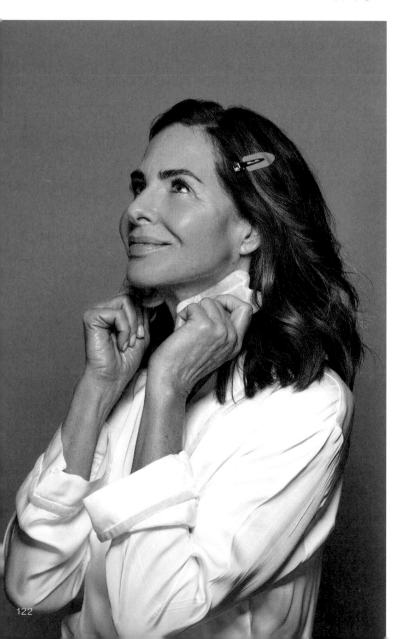

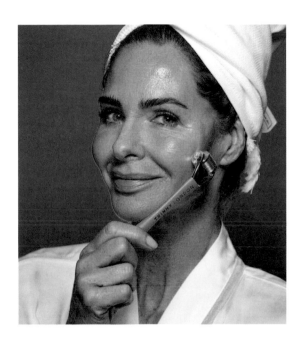

Micro-needling

This might be a scary idea to many, but it is an incredible treatment that can help with scarring, pigmentation, sagging skin and fine lines. In clinic, it will have a greater impact than doing it at home partly because the needle depth will be greater. I would not recommend a roller with a needle more than 0.5 millimetre in depth for at home treatments. It is rolled over the skin, which creates 'micro channels' to allow the product you put on to be absorbed deeply. This also stimulates the skin, rebuilding collagen and elastin. I do this once or twice a week.

How to micro-needle at home:

- Rollers come with needles in a range of diameters. If it is your first time, start with 0.5mm needles and light strokes.

- Remember to replace the roller heads after about 10 uses, as the needles become blunt and stop being effective.

- Clean the roller head after use.

- Make sure the skin is well cleansed.

- Avoid the sensitive eye area.

- This is best followed with a non-irritating serum, like a hyluronic acid or peptide, and avoid anything with fragrance.

This is not good for people with sensitive skin, acne, eczema or rosacea. This can be used for acne scarring. Always seek the advice of a dermatologist or start with an in-salon treatment.

Common skin issues

Let's look at this from another angle. What steps can you take to combat specific skin problems?

If you have dry skin

The first thing I always ask women who tell me they have dry skin is: do you have dry skin or dehydrated skin? Dry skin is naturally lacking in oil. Your skin isn't moisturising itself from the inside. If you have dry skin you've probably had it your whole life, or following a hormonal change like the menopause.

Dehydrated skin is skin that is lacking water. It's caused by external factors like not drinking enough water, washing in too-hot water, using harsh skincare that strips the oils or the environment, like central heating or spending a lot of time in a hot, windy climate.

A test is to give up tea and coffee for three days and drink as much water as you can - up to three litres. If on the fourth day, your skin feels less tight, then dehydration is definitely part of the problem. People with dry skin often think that if they just find the right moisturiser then it will solve everything and they overlook the importance of exfoliation. A build up of dead skin cells will make your face feel dull and rough, plus they will be blocking the serum and moisturiser you use from getting in. Get your exfoliation right and you'll feel the energy and vibrancy of your skin.

- AHAs (introduce slowly) or PHAs if you have sensitive skin
- Ceramides
- Hyaluronic acid

If you have oily skin

For some, the sebaceous glands produce too much sebum - the natural oils that keep our skin soft and comfortable - leaving us with anything from shiny skin, especially around the t-zone, to oily skin, which can trap bacteria, causing breakouts. However, it's not all bad. If you have oily skin, fine lines and wrinkles are likely to be less of an issue for you as your skin doesn't dry out the same.

Hormones can be a big factor for people with oily skin (and acne), which is why it's often associated with our teenage years but can also come back around with the menopause, when our hormone levels change again. Diet also affects sebum production and it can be triggered by specific foods, so keep a food diary to give you insight. Hot and humid climates can be a factor, as can stress.

You are looking for products that can help normalise sebum production, so you glow rather than shine. It sounds obvious, but the main thing is to avoid adding extra oil to your face. So you particularly want to look out for gels. It's a myth that you don't need to moisturise if you have oily skin - oily skin can still lack water. Just look for something lightweight, like a hyaluronic acid.

- Salicylic acid (a BHA - use cautiously at first if you have sensitive skin)

- Niacinamide

- Hyaluronic acid

If you have combination skin

Combination skin is where you have excess oil across your T-zone but are prone to dry, tight skin across your cheeks. It's very common but can present a challenge to deal with, as you can feel like you are constantly changing your routine, trying to find balance. The right cleanser that doesn't strip the oil but cleans the pores is important. It's fine to use AHAs to target the oilier areas and discourage blocked pores but do use moisturiser all over.

- AHAs

- Vitamin C - though carefully at first and not everyday

- Hyaluronic acid

If you have sensitive skin

A lot of things come under the umbrella of 'sensitive skin' so it's important to first ask 'sensitive, how?' Do you get redness, rosacea (see right), itching, rashes, sore and tight skin? Many of us find that hormones and periods of stress exacerbate skin issues. The key here is to really listen to your skin and notice if something is causing irritation. You may want to go back to basics with a cleanser and moisturiser that works for you, stick to the routine and then introduce other things - like a serum - one at a time. It's still important to exfoliate your skin in a way that's right for you so you get that new skin showing through.

- PHAs
- Ceramides
- Peptides
- Azelaic acid

If you have acne

Spots are caused when a pore is blocked with a plug of sebum and skin cells. Bacteria can get in and cause inflammation. This can be treated and often prevented with topical skincare. Acne, however, is an inflammatory skin condition linked to hormones.

If you use harsh products, you'll make your skin worse. You need kindness and calm. We are supposed to produce sebum, and we have a microbiome on our faces of yeasts and good bacteria, and we don't want to upset this balance. First, try to soothe the inflammation, as you will then be able to tolerate stronger retinoids, BHAs and niacinamide, which can help long term. Start with the basics and always double cleanse. Take a product break and use a light, non-oil based moisturiser for a few days.

The key questions to ask: are you changing your pillow frequently; do you tie your hair back when you sleep; are you avoiding sugars that cause inflammation; and if you have back acne, do you wash the residual shampoo/conditioner off your skin?

If your acne is making you miserable, then do seek medical advice. I have absolutely been there and there are things you can do.

- Glycolic or salicylic acid

- Retinoids

- Humectant moisturisers

- Niacinamide

- Prescription drugs (e.g. Roaccutane)

Lots of us suffer from tiny white or flesh coloured 'milk spots' just under the skin called Milia. Rather than pus, as with a blemish, they contain a build up of keratin, a protein. Absolutely do not squeeze them (especially not around the sensitive eye area) but rather make sure you double cleanse, exfoliate in a way that works for the rest of your skin and use a retinoid (although again, not too close to your eyes). There are in-clinic treatments that can really help, but you must maintain this by exfoliating.

If you have rosacea

This condition causes skin to look flushed and even feel like it's burning. Anyone can suffer from it. If your skin stings sometimes when you go from hot to cold environments or after eating certain foods, it may be rosacea. There is no exact cause and no catch-all treatment. It's about finding a way to manage it. Avoid washing in hot water or using scrubs, take care of the skin's natural barrier and see a dermatologist if it is causing you discomfort.

- Ceramide

- Niacinamide

- Azelaic acid

If you are peri/menopausal

When your hormones are changing your skin changes too. You might find you are suddenly suffering from acne or your skin is drying out. As our skin ages, collagen and elastin reduces and our skin eventually produces fewer lipids - although, as our oestrogen levels drop we can actually see an increase in oils in the skin, which is one of the reasons we can experience breakouts.

- Peptides

- Hyaluronic acid

- Ceramide

If you have hyperpigmentation

This is an umbrella term, where patches of the skin become darker, with different conditions sitting beneath it. It can be caused by sun damage and hormones (including taking birth control and pregnancy), or follow skin damage like bad breakouts or wounds. Always wear an SPF, particularly as you approach the menopause. If you are ever concerned that a mark might be a sign of something more sinister, always get it checked out.

- Vitamin C

- AHAs

- Retinoids (at night)

How to read an INCI list

Pronounced 'Inkey' (it took me years to know this), this refers to the ingredients listed on the packaging of a product. Brands don't have to say how much of each ingredient has been used, but the list is always in descending order of percentage for anything above 1%, below this they can be listed in any order. Therefore, if the product is highlighting a specific ingredient, you should expect to see this in the top half of the list.

Generally, anything under fragrance will be an incredibly small amount of the ingredient. Of course, just because an ingredient is used in a low concentration, that doesn't always mean it won't be effective. Some active ingredients are effective in very low percentages. It is a good way to get a sense of how much is in the serum or cream you have in your hand, though. If the product is claiming it uses ingredients on the pack, then you want to see those ingredient names as high up the ingredient list as possible.

A very common skincare ingredient is phenoxyethanol, a preservative, and you will see this in many products on the shelf. A useful rule of thumb is that this can only be used in concentrations of up to 1 per cent in skincare, so anything that is below this on the INCI list is less than 1 per cent of the product. Again, this is not always a terrible thing, but handy to know as a point of quick reference for those other ingredient amounts.

Also, near the INCI list, you'll often see a symbol that looks like a jar with a lid hovering above and a number (this stands for the number of months) followed by an M (month). This indicates the shelf life of a product once it's been opened. It doesn't mean that it will immediately become 'bad' or start irritating your skin on the exact day, say six months after cracking the seal - it just might not be particularly effective any more. The most important one to keep an eye on is probably SPF creams, as they typically have a 12 month shelf life coupled with high consequences for your skin if they're not working.

Tired eyes

Puffy eyes and dark circles are the bane of so many of our lives and I am asked how to improve both often.

If you have puffy eyes

At night, when your body is still, fluid can build up. Sleeping face down or lying very flat can make this worse, so try to elevate your head. When we eat too many high-salt foods or drink sugary alcoholic drinks, our bodies hold on to extra water in an attempt to flush them out. Alcohol is also the enemy of a good night's sleep. Hormones can also cause bloating in your face, not just your stomach, around the time of your period.

- Improve your sleep

- Reduce your salt and alcohol intake

- Massage your face in the morning (see page 119)

If you have dark circles

We have natural fat pads beneath our eyes, which for most people, aren't very visible when we're younger. As we age, our skin loses its elasticity and plumpness, meaning the pads become more prominent. Our skin becomes thinner, and the blood vessels that surround our eyes become more apparent too.

You may also suffer from hyperpigmentation, which is caused by an overproduction of the protein melanin. It can appear around the eyes where the skin is thinner.

- Drink plenty of water

- Double cleanse AM and PM

- Check your iron and B12 levels with a blood test

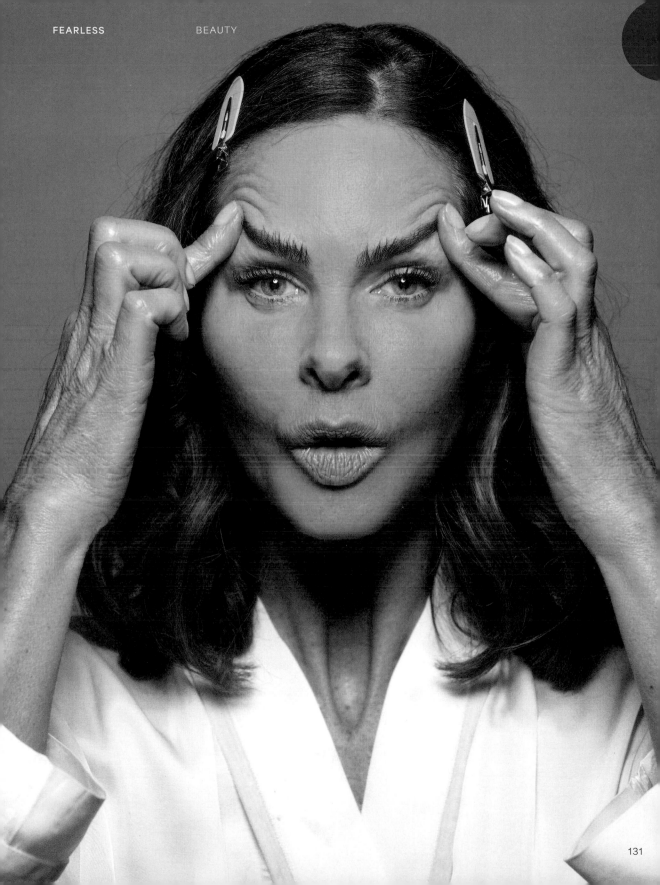

Skincare and tweakments

It's important to understand what you can reasonably expect from a product and when, even if it contains the very best in active ingredients, its effectiveness will end. Beauty marketing would like us to believe that the latest product will work some sort of miracle, leaving us disappointed and annoyed when we spend money on something that doesn't deliver.

We all have things we like more and less about our faces and our bodies. If something really bothers you – like dark circles always making you feel drained when you look in the mirror, no matter how much sleep you've had, for example – you will probably be prepared to spend more time and more money on addressing that.

No one should feel they have to have in-salon treatment, tweakments or more. If you can dab a bit of undereye concealer on your dark circles and not think about them anymore then that's great. It's all about personal choice and feeling empowered and informed to make the decisions that are right for us, to get the results we want to see.

If you decide to opt for a cosmetic procedure then you must, must do your research, consult a specialist and find a good practitioner whose work you can see examples of. This is not somewhere to cut corners. And always make sure you have a realistic understanding of any downtime. Seek out testimonials from a range of people who have had the tweakment or procedure – don't just rely on what the clinic or salon has posted on their website.

Here, I have asked the brilliant Alice Hart-Davis to give us some more information on the treatments and results you can achieve whichever option you select. Alice has been reporting on (and trying out) cosmetic procedures for 25 years and is the founder of thetweakmentsguide.com, an online treasure trove of trusted advice on cosmetic procedures, practitioners and how to get the best results.

Skin ageing

Where	What	What to expect
At home	Retinoids and peptides	Smoother, firmer skin
In salon	Advanced facial with microneedling; LED light therapy	Fine lines smoothed and less noticeable. Healthier, stronger skin
At the dermatologist	Botox; filler; radiofrequency microneedling	Softened frown lines and crow's feet, better contours of cheeks and jawline, smoother stronger skin
Cosmetic surgery	Facelift	Big impact that can last up to 10 years. Expensive, lengthy recovery. Best value procedure is often an upper eye lift

Sagging neck/jowls

Where	What	What to expect
At home	Micro electric current through a device (NuFace/FaceGym Pro)	A gentle tightening of the muscles, if done 3 times a week
In salon	Radiofrequency microneedling or ultrasound skin tightening	A day's downtime. RF needling needs three monthly treatments
At the dermatologist	Threads, fat-dissolving injections or fat-freezing for double chins	Threads will lift the cheeks back up and make skin more taut but only last 8–18 months
Cosmetic surgery	Neck or lower face lift	Refined jawline and defined neck contours, lasts 10 years

Acne scarring

Where	What	What to expect
At home	Retinol and micro-needling	A gentle softness to the look of the scarring
In salon	Fractional radiofrequency	Gently smoother looking skin
At the dermatologist	CO2 laser	A noticeable improvement to the skin. 2–4 weeks downtime

Melasma/age spots/pigmentation

Where	What	What to expect
At home	Vitamin C and vigilant use of SPF 50	Difference in small age spots. Melasma will be less obvious
In salon	LED light, IPL (age spots) Cosmelan (melasma)	Total removal, conditional upon consistent use of SPF 50
At the dermatologist	Prescription skincare; Pico lasers (safe for all skin types)	Reduction/ removal of brown spots and patchy pigmentation

Under eye bags

Where	What	What to expect
At home	Eye cream with caffeine, lymph-drainage massage	Small reduction of puffiness and eye bags
In salon	Professional lymph-drainage massage, microcurrent facials	Some flattening of eye bags and refining of face contours
At the dermatologist	Radiofrequency microneedling	Tighter skin, reduced bagging
Cosmetic surgery	Lower blepharoplasty (eye lift)	Smoother, fresher-looking, de-bagged under-eyes

ASK YOURSELF

1 Do you feel you can't be bothered to do a full skincare routine in the morning?

2 Do you have a nightime skincare routine?

3 How much water do you actually drink?

4 Do you think what you eat has an impact on your skin?

5 On a level of 1-10 how stressed are you each day?

6 Did you wake up one day and think, what the f*** happened?!

CHALLENGE YOURSELF

1 Your morning skincare routine should take you 5 minutes. I hope everyone can take that time for themselves each morning. Please, just try it for 1 week and see if you notice the difference to your skin.

2 Since you have been able to identify your skin type (see page 16) and your issues (see pages 124-128), it will be easier to find the products that work for you and avoid wasting your money on the wrong items. Day 1 buy yourself the correct serum and, before you buy anything else, use it for 2 weeks to see the changes. Introduce each new product one at a time and keep track of the improvement.

3 For great skin you must drink a minimum of two litres of water a day. This will make a huge impact on your skin and body health. I always lie to myself on this one.

4 Salt, sugar and alcohol have been proven to have a negative impact on the skin. It can lead to puffiness around the face. Keep a food diary for a week. At the end, look at everything together and question what proportion of your diet includes excess amounts of these inflammatory foods and drinks. Think about how you could very simply reduce your intake throughout the week.

5 For a week measure your stress levels, by rating each day from 1 (minimal) to 10 (extremely high). If you are above 5 most days, there will be a damaging level of the stress hormone cortisol in your body. Reduce this stress by exercising and meditating, which have been proven to help bring these levels down.

6 Don't panic. We have all been there. There are solutions. Go back to the beginning of this chapter and follow the things you can do now to help your skin feel at its best.

THE INGREDIENT LIST

Exfoliating acid family

If putting 'acid' on your face sounds like a terrible idea, don't worry, it's not. These liquid exfoliants help to remove dead skin cells that would otherwise clog your skin and make it look dull. Generally, liquid exfoliants can be put on the skin and left on. A strong acid peel can only be performed by a dermatologist.

AHAs

Alpha-hydroxy acids, including glycolic, lactic and malic acid. Their molecules are smaller than the other acids so they can penetrate more deeply into the skin.

What do they do?

Dissolve the bonds that hold dead skin cells to the surface, to reveal a brighter, clearer complexion.

Target hyperpigmentation and dull skin.

Who should use them?

Anyone who wants to restore glow to their skin with fine lines.

Particularly those with dull, dry skin who really need to clear those dead skin cells and whatever moisturiser they use still makes them feel dry.

Not for those with very sensitive skin.

When should you use them?

In the PM, as they can increase the skin's sensitivity to the sun. Use after cleansing.

You may want to start with just a 2-3 times a week while your skin gets used to them.

If you use retinoids you might want to alternate nights.

BHAs

Beta-hydroxy acids. The one most commonly used in skincare is salicylic acid or willow bark.

What do they do?

Salicylic acids primary benefit is as an exfoliant, helping shed dead skin. Because it has the ability to penetrate and exfoliate inside the pore as well as on the surface of skin, it's especially effective for reducing breakouts – including blackheads and whiteheads.

Who should use them?

Anyone with a combination, oily or blemish-prone complexion.

When should you use them?

In the PM, after cleansing as they can make your skin more light sensitive.

Use a couple of times a week and not with retinoids, while your skin builds up tolerance. Increase if this feels beneficial.

PHAs

Polyhydroxy acids such as gluconolactone and lactobionic. The molecules of this acid are larger so they are slower to penetrate into the skin and are therefore more gentle. They are still effective way of exfoliating and are less likely to cause irritation.

What do they do?

PHAs exfoliate and hydrate. They hydrate the skin and are powerful antioxidants making them perfect for sensitive and dehydrated skin. The exfoliation process boosts the skin's glow and radiance.

Who should use them?

First-time acid users, or anyone with more sensitive skin.

When should you use them?

AM or PM. They are gentler, don't increase sun sensitivity and they play well with other ingredients.

Ceramides

What do they do?
Ceramides bond our skin cells together, sort of like the mortar between bricks. They are an important part of a healthy skin barrier and help lock in moisture.

Who should use them?
Anyone with dry skin or irritated skin.

When should you use them?
Ceramides usually come in the form of a serum or moisturiser and can be applied AM or PM.

Hyaluronic acid

What does it do?
Although it's also called an 'acid' it's very different to the liquid exfoliators we talk about above. It's a hydrator, a humectant that hold up to 1,000 times its weight in moisture inside your skin.

Who should use them?
All skin types can benefit but those with dehydrated skin will see the most improvement. If you want to get technical, hydrolyzed hyaluronic acid has the smallest molecules and will likely penetrate the skin more deeply.

When should you use them?
Any time. It plays nicely with other ingredients, just make sure you use it before anything oily so it can penetrate the skin. Only avoid if you are going somewhere very dry, like on a plane or going to an arrid climate, as it can then start to suck water from the skin. These are best in a serum, not moisturiser.

Niacinamide

What does it do?

Niacinamide is a form of vitamin B3 and a powerful, hard-working active. It has a number of different benefits. Including:

- Targeting pigmentation to brighten and even skin tone.

- Boosting hydration by supporting the skin structure and improving the barrier function.

- Has soothing properties.

- Balancing the production of sebum, preventing breakouts, so useful for oily, spot prone skin.

- Reducing the signs of ageing by increasing the energy level of the cells.

Who should use them?

Almost everyone will benefit from incorporating it into their routine, but it's especially good for spot prone or stressed skin.

When should you use them?

AM or PM. Best used after cleansing or exfoliating in a leave-on product like a serum or moisturiser.

Peptides

Types of peptides

Peptides are short chains of amino acids that are the building blocks of proteins. The proteins we most care about in skincare are collagen, elastin and keratin, as they are responsible for the plumpness and elasticity of our skin. However, their molecules are large and won't be absorbed into our skin if we put them in a cream. Peptides, meanwhile, can get into the skin, where they can do a number of jobs.

Signal peptides: send messages to encourage the production of proteins like collagen and elastin.

Neurotransmitter inhibitor peptides: help block the release of chemicals that cause the muscle contractions of expression lines. They work in a similar way to Botox, although the effect is subtler, softening existing lines and preventing new ones from forming.

Carrier peptides: help to transport elements that help the formation of proteins (like collagen and elastin) to where they need to be.

Enzyme inhibitor peptides: help to prevent the breakdown of existing collagen and elastin.

Who should use them?

Peptides are effective at a very low percentage and don't tend to irritate the skin, so they are fine even if you have sensitive skin. They become more important as our skin ages.

When should you use them?

Best used after exfoliating in a leave-on product like a serum or moisturiser. They can be used at any time of day.

Vitamin C

There are so many vitamin Cs in the market... It's something I have used in my routine for over 25 years, and an essential I would never be without.

What does it do?

Vitamin C or 'ascorbic acid' is one of the most important and beneficial multitasking skincare ingredients. It:

- Is an antioxidant. It protects and shields the skin from free radical damage caused by things like pollution, UV and stress (it sacrifices itself to save your skin from damage).

- Brightens dullness.

- Helps fade and prevent visible pigmentation.

- Encourages collagen production as Vitamin C is involved in this process. The collagen protein is naturally required for plump, bouncy skin.

Who should use them?

Everyone, with all skin types, from the age of 30 should start incorporating a vitamin C into your morning routine (at the serum step) to help slow down those signs of ageing that quickly catch up with you in your forties and fifties.

There are different types of vitamin C and it comes in different strengths so it can be confusing. The key is to find the right form and strength that suits your skin type and goals.

When should you use them?

In the morning. Vitamin C does some of its best work during the day, flexing its antioxidant abilities to support your SPF and shield skin from damaging free radicals. When you're using your vitamin C in the morning always follow it with moisturiser, if needed, and without fail an SPF!

There are new forms of vitamin C being developed all the time. Vitamin C has proven antioxidant activity at low levels, however I would suggest if you are looking for a good vitamin C to protect your skin from damage during the day, my rule of thumb is to use a vitamin C with at least 10-15% concentration. If your goal is to reduce stubborn pigmentation or treat melasma, higher levels of up to 20-30% may be necessary.

Water soluble ones are generally suitable for all skin types:

L-Ascorbic acid

What to use	This needs to be at a concentration of 8-20% to be effective. It can be bought on its own as a powder or combined with an antioxidant, like ferulic acid, in a product.
Pros	• The most potent form of vitamin C. • Relatively cheap to buy. • Best for targeting stubborn pigmentation/age spots.
Cons	• It is the least stable form and reacts with air and light, so needs to be stored correctly (in a cool, dark place). • Due to its low pH, it can cause irritation on the skin. • You should take care when applying near the eye area.

3-O-Ethyl ascorbic acid

What to use Can be used up to 30%. The pH4-5.5 is close to the skins natural pH level.

Pros
- Good for all skin types.
- Good at boosting collagen, reducing pigmentation and brightening skin.
- It doesn't get to work until it has fully absorbed, so it is less likely to upset the skin.

Cons
- Those with sensitive skin may find it causes irritation when used in higher percentages.

Sodium ascorbyl phosphate

Pros
- Best for oily/blemish prone skin.
- A good everyday antioxidant.
- For those with acne, it works well with blemish-busting salicylic acid.
- It is more stable so less likely to cause irritation.

Cons
- This is a salt version of ascorbic acid, so it will be slower acting.
- It is generally not used at higher concentrations.

Magnesium ascorbyl phosphate

Pros
- One of the best for brightening.
- Salt form of ascorbic acid so less irritating.
- More stable than L-Ascorbic acid.

Cons
- This is another salt version of ascorbic acid, containing magnesium salt, so it will be slower acting.
- It is generally not used at higher concentrations.

Ascorbyl glucoside

Pros
- It is water soluble, so remains stable at a range of pH levels.
- Considered a gentler formula.
- It is good for sensitive skin.

Cons
- Less effective than most other forms.

Ascorbyl palmitate

Pros
- Has antioxidant properties.

Cons
- Mostly used to stop ingredients in a formula from oxidising.
- Has little of the benefits of vitamin C.

Oil soluble vitamin C feels oilier and is generally better for drier skin types. They can penetrate the skin up to 50x faster than L-ascorbic acid so are considered the next generation in vitamin C technology. On the ingredients list, I look for the name with 'tetra' in it. This indicates it is oil soluble. Two of the main ingredients are:

Ascorbyl tetraisopalmitate

What to use	Used in concentrations of 20% when targeting hyperpigmentation.
Pros	• Good for drier skin types. • Excellent antioxidant properties. • Excellent at stopping collagen breakdown.
Cons	• Formulas may not suit oilier skin types. • It can be too strong for sensitive skin.

Tetrahexyldecyl ascorbate

What to use	Effective at 0.1% but can be used at 5-30% to target hyperpigmentation or melasma.
Pros	• Good for drier skin types. • Excellent at stopping collagen breakdown.
Cons	• Formulas may not suit oilier skin. • At higher percentages, it may be too strong for sensitive skin.

The vitamin A family (retinoids)

I'm giving this essential active a section to itself as of all the ingredients on the market, retinoid can be very effective. Retinoic acid has been the gold standard in tackling skin ageing since the 1980's. You can only get it on prescription so the cosmetic industry has spent decades trying to match its powerful effects in cosmetic forms. Here's a simple overview to help you navigate this complex world.

What do they do?

- Reduce fine lines and wrinkles by jump-starting dwindling production of collagen, helping skin to replenish lost stocks.
- Helps to clear breakouts and prevent new ones from forming by speeding up skin cell turnover.
- Makes skin appear brighter and more even in tone.
- Fades pigmentation over time.
- Prevents future age spots, blocking transportation of melanin.

Who should use them?

- Anyone who wants to treat fine lines.
- Anyone with sebaceous skin who is prone to spots.
- Those with acne.

When should you use them?

Every day in the evening, after exfoliating, letting it sink in before you put anything over the top, unless:

- You are using a high-strength retinoid.
- You have just started using an AHA or BHA.
- You have very sensitive skin. Start slowly in this case.
- Avoid retinoids if you are pregnant or breastfeeding.

There are a number of members of the retinoid family and they are used as an ingredient in cosmetic skincare in slightly different ways by brands. What is right for you will depend a lot on how sensitive your skin is and what you want to get out of the product.

Very strong retinoic acids are sometimes prescribed by doctors as a treatment for acne (this is where it started as a skincare ingredient). Unless you need them, I don't think prescription-strength retinoids are a good idea as they are harsh and your skin will go through a process of peeling and flaking.

If you are using a stronger retinoid you may want to use it a couple of times a week, rather than every night. It may take a couple of weeks for your skin to get used to, so listen to your skin. If it feels dry and sore, perhaps you need to try something else.

Some serums and creams boast high levels of retinoids but more isn't always more here. Because it is an irritant, these may contain ingredients that soothe the skin too, to counteract the irritation. A lower strength can still actively improve your skin, without needing other ingredients to soothe the powerful retinoids.

You can use retinoids on your neck but bear in mind the skin tends to be more sensitive here and you will need to make sure it is rubbed in properly.

You can spend a lot of money on the very best retinals and retinoates, and the technology is developing all the time. But you don't need to jump in at the high end. Find a decent high street brand and see how you get on. You can always invest more later, particularly as you get older and you experience more fine lines.

Here is a run-down of the types of retinoids you will encounter in cosmetic skincare:

Retinyl palmitate

Pros	• Widely available. • In many less expensive skincare products. • Can be used by those with sensitive skin who are irritated by other forms.
Cons	• Not a very effective form. Unlikely to give good results.

Retinaldehyde (sometimes shortened to retinal)

Pros	• Absorbed and used more effectively by the skin in this form. • Less likely to irritate the skin.
Cons	• Mainly found in more expensive products.

HPRetinoate

Pros	• Very efficient. • Unlikely to cause irritation.
Cons	• New technology that's only just coming into skincare. • Likely to be very expensive.

Granactive retinol (hydroxypinacolone retinoate)

Pros	• A relatively new form of retinoid that binds directly onto retinoic recepters in the skin and switches them on.
	• Low irritation, fast acting.
Cons	• New technology that's only just coming into skincare.

Retinol

Pros	• One of the first most powerful cosmetic ingredients available.
Cons	• It is not very stable in light and air so needs to be formulated extremely well.
	• It can often be irritating to the skin as it starts to oxidise on the surface.
	• Undergoes a 2-step conversion in the skin, so some of its effectiveness can be lost in this process.

Bear in mind that a 1% retinyl palmitate is not as strong and slower to work than a 0.3% retinal, because this form is less effective on the skin

HAIR

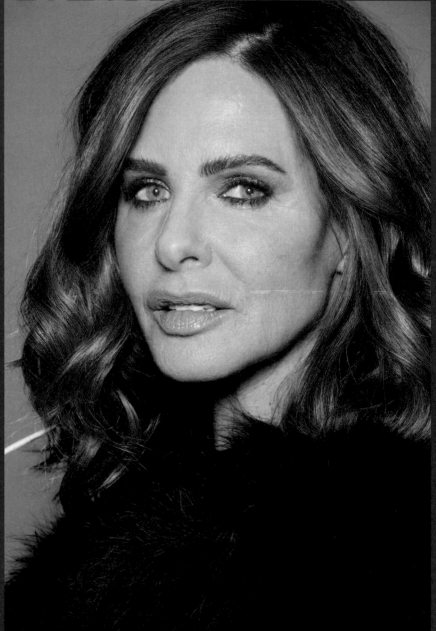

IS EVERYTHING

Hair

Isn't it interesting how when we feel our most confident we don't worry about our hair, and when we feel stuck or unsure who we want to be we are more likely to go for a drastic change?

Having a great haircut that brings definition to our face makes us feel assured - our style and makeup comes together more effortlessly. And when we haven't given our hair enough attention recently we can feel like we are fading into the background. So embracing a style that works for you is important, but so is caring for it between cuts.

We need to be kind to our hair and listen to it, just like we do our skin. You wouldn't spend money on a facial and then not bother with a skincare routine. We should think about hair in a similar way, as hair, skin and makeup are all very connected. It's hard to feel really good about one if you have been neglecting another.

Our hair changes as we go down the path of life just like our skin does - and not just in terms of going grey. That's perfectly natural, though it does present us with new challenges.

Hair, skin and makeup are all connected

Hair for the decades

As we go down the path of life, we will likely try many different styles and possibly a few different colours too. Your hair is a great way to change up your style and refresh your look.

Twenties

You might experiment with dye (don't forget your colour code – see page 15). Hair straighteners will damage your hair, so do use heat protection spray to maintain its condition going forward.

Thirties

This is the time to up your maintainance and trim between your cuts (it will be cheaper than a full cut).

Forties

You will now know the time, money and energy you are prepared to put into maintaining your hair, so stick to your strengths.

Fifties

The menopause can have a significant impact on hair – the change will vary and depend on whether you take HRT. This is when hair that once felt healthy edges into brittle and dry. Whatever the natural texture, adding moisture and encouraging shine will prevent it looking dull. Do take supplements (see pages 91–93).

Sixties and beyond

Having a cut that frames your face will give you structure, which, as we age, is needed as we lose bone, muscle and collagen.

The non-essential essentials

Always remember to be kind to your hair. Just as using too many skincare products can lead to upsetting the balance of our faces and stripping away the natural oils, throwing everything at our hair and then blasting it with heat is not going to give us the shiny, happy hair we want.

1 Hair masks

These are great for dry hair, frizzy ends, or if you bleach your hair. You can do this every 2-4 weeks. I find the pre-wash mask is less heavy on my hair, so I use Josh Wood's Miracle Mask.

2 Product cleansing shampoo

I use this every few weeks. They are great for getting rid of product build up that can make your hair look flakey, dull and flat. If needed, use one that is suitable for colour-treated hair.

3 Dry shampoo

Try spraying it in before you go to bed so it can work at night, rather than trying to rub it all in. If you have very thin, fine hair try a product that's a bit lighter and more subtle.

4 Hand cream

Yes, hand cream. It contains similar ingredients to hair finishing cream. If you are suffering from frizzy ends, moisturising your hands and very lightly stroking the residue over them will help.

5 Heat protection spray

Please always use heat protection spray, it's worth it. The need for our hair to always look good prevents us acknowledging the long term damage that heat can do. Learning how to blow dry your hair or to work with the curl not against it might be better options than using hair straighteners every day.

Hair loss

This is a serious concern for lots of women and I don't think we talk about it enough. It can be caused by a range of factors, some hormonal, some to do with stress and illness (I experienced hair loss after having Covid and during the menopause). Though most experts agree that these factors all come down to inflammation in the body. If you are experiencing hair loss then it's important to try to understand the underlying cause. For some women, this may be as simple as not having enough iron in the diet – so getting this checked by your GP is a good place to start.

Always remember to be kind to your hair. Just as using too many skincare products can lead to upsetting the balance of our faces and stripping away the natural oils, throwing everything at our hair and then blasting it with heat is not going to give us the shiny, happy hair we want.

There are shampoos that promise to reduce hair loss, although all they can do is slow down the rate your hair is shed from the follicle; they won't stimulate new growth. If your hair is mainly thinning around your temples then there are root coverup products that you can use to subtly fill this gap, such as Color Wow, which I find make a big difference to restoring the natural proportions of my face. Weaves, extensions, braiding and simply pulling your hair back tightly with harsh bands can cause thinning here, so it's about balancing short-term gain against possible long-term consequences. I also take Biotin supplements, and I do believe they help.

Your best hair colour

A lot of women colour their hair a shade that doesn't quite fit with their natural skin and eye tone. I have done this more than once. I look back at photos of when I was having a red hair moment and see that it was just too warm for me!

The temptation to experiment with our hair is strong for many of us. But whatever you want to do, I would say: never lose sight of your natural hair colour. Even if you think it's boring, it's yours; the fact is, no one is born with a hair colour that doesn't suit their skin and eyes. If you try to go completely against it, it puts you out of kilter. You will find it harder to know what make up and clothes work well for you.

The importance of eye colour

One test is to look at the relationship between your current hair colour and your eye colour. Put a chunk of hair next to your eye. When they are in harmony, your eyes will pop; if your hair takes away from your eye colour, making things feel murkier, you don't have it quite right yet.

The other thing to consider is the relationship between your skin and your hair colour – do they sit naturally together or do you feel they may be pulling how you look in different directions? Again, they should always work together.

Try someone new

If you have been going to the same hairdresser for years, then do ask yourself if they are taking into account how your face and hair (and perhaps style and personality) is changing, or whether they just do the same old colour every time. If so, it might be time to get a fresh take from someone else. (Though I do know that finding a good hairdresser can be a little like the search for the perfect romantic partner ... ask friends who you think have great hair where they go and always pop in for a consultation before you commit.)

When is it time to embrace the grey...?

Younger women, stay with me here. You don't know when you might start to see grey hairs and it's good to know what lies ahead. Grey hair can be liberating and very beautiful, and for others, going grey is unimaginable (me!).

A lot of women decide to go grey when their colour maintenance becomes too time consuming or boring, particularly with roots that show quickly. Or their original colour is now too harsh and silvery grey is a look they are ready to embrace.

The hardest way to make the change is to grow out the colour, as it takes perseverance and you might not feel good about your hair for a while. Getting some grey lights put in can help and some people chose to go blonde first to ease the transition. This is not an option for everyone of course, and if you have never had very light hair before it can feel like a bit of a shock to the system.

Your colour palette

Grey is by nature a cooler shade, so your wardrobe is cool it will be less of an adjustment. However, if you have a darker skin tone and you are a warm/neutral or warm then this will take a bit more thought. You might find that some darker tones now wash you out and your best neutrals - navies, burgundies, greys - change. The way you do your makeup will be different too.

The colour and condition of your hair

Grey hair can look dirty or lifted. It's rare that naturally grey hair won't need any tending at all. The subtlest blue rinse or a purple shampoo may hold the key to bringing life and avoid it looking dull and flat. If your hair is very white then look into blue shampoos. As always, it is about light and movement. Give some time and attention to getting the right cut and maintaining the condition and you will feel great about your new grey hair.

50 SHADES

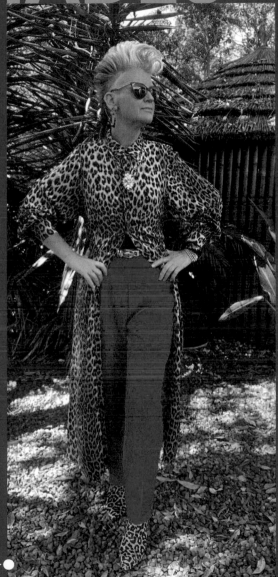

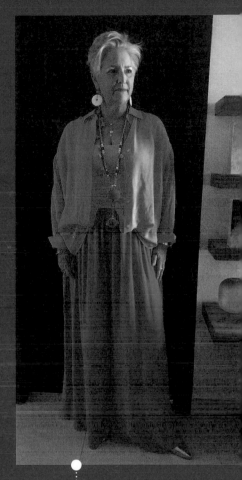

CARRIE

LISA

OF
GREY?

A SOURCE

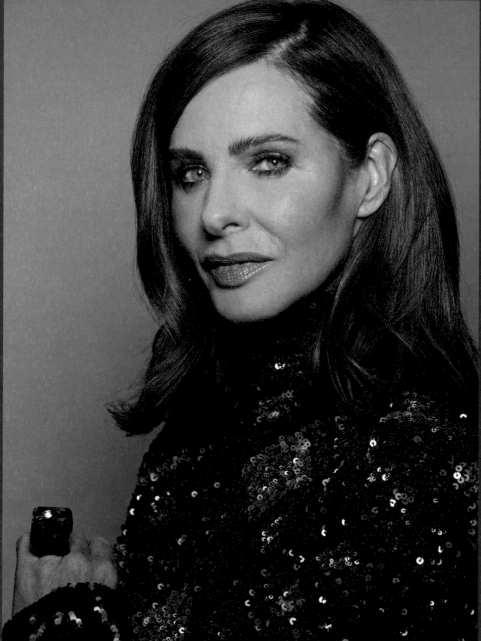

OF JOY

Makeup

Makeup means that if I wake up feeling tired, I don't have to look at a drained face in the mirror all day. I can take an undereye concealer, blusher and a bright lip and in minutes I look - and therefore feel - more awake, ready to face the day.

When I want to wear a fabulous strong colour, by paying attention to how I do my makeup, I can make sure that it doesn't dominate me, that I don't get lost behind it.

And when I am heading out in the evening, by giving myself the time do a smokey eye, I give myself the space to take a moment to catch up from my busy day and instantly feel more confident.

Sometimes we can get bored of our makeup look. We can become stuck in a rut, lose our confidence or feel like we don't know what works for us any more. In this part of the book, I am going to try to give you the tools and help you to feel inspired to elevate your look and try something new.

A small discovery can make a big difference

The tools

Whether you apply your makeup with a brush, a sponge or your fingers largely comes down to personal preference.

I prefer cream-based blushers, bronzers and eyeshades. They are so much easier to blend, they stay where they are put and they happily make friends with your skin. Powders are more likely to cake or collect unhelpfully in your lines. Creams are very easy to apply with your fingers, though for a more polished look, a brush brings precision and will help you blend once it's on your face. Powders generally need a brush.

The six brushes I use all the time are:

- **An angled contour brush** for eye colour and heavier concealer. It gives a softer finish and stops you putting too much on (I use fingers for lighter concealer under my eyes)

- **A fluffy tapered brush** for bronzer and blusher, if I want to be really targeted in where it's going

- **A large domed brush** to blend my base and ensure it's all even

- **A dense buffer brush** to blend

- **A lip brush** will add softer definition than a liner

- **A narrow angled brush** to add eye colour to my lash line

I also like to use a sponge to apply and blend my base. However, this is something that must be washed every day. If you don't think you will do this, then don't buy a sponge.

You must wash your brushes regularly too. You can buy special brush cleaner (which sometimes doesn't need water, so good if you're on the go) but mild shampoo or a gentle hand soap is perfectly fine. The average makeup brush contains more bacteria than our mobile phones or even the notoriously grubby London Underground. You do not want to be putting that brush into your precious products or onto your beautifully cleansed face. And consider treating your make up bag to a regular clean, too.

The essentials

This is something I am asked about a lot. To me, this is the basic kit. If you have these things to hand, you are always good to go.

1 **BB cream/tinted moisturiser with SPF**
This will wake up tired skin or smooth out an uneven skin tone.

2 **A brilliant concealer and undereye**
It's worth having both. You want a lightweight concealer that won't crease and something denser to cover redness.

3 **Mascara**
Along with a brush to comb it through and get rid of clumps.

4 **Blusher**
Has the power to bring life to your complexion.

5 **Eyebrow gel**
Eyebrows bring structure and definition to the face.

6 **Eye shade deeper than your skin tone**
This will frame your eye, creating a shape around your eye socket.

7 **Lip shade to enhance your lip colour**
An easy-to-wear shade that gives you that no makeup look.

8 **Tweezers**
The older you get, the more you will need these for rogue hairs!

The non-essential essentials

Just like the non-essential essentials that elevate the staples in your wardrobe (see page 243), these are the extras that will give you a lift and bring your makeup to life.

1   **Contour and highlighter**
Much easier to use than you might think, they bring definition and a radiant glow to the party.

2   **Brow pencil**
To bring strength to your brows - particularly if they are thin.

3   **Eye pencil**
Not all of us suit a noticeable line across the eyelid, but something subtle on the lower and upper lash line can bring focus.

4   **Eye shade that enhances your eye colour**
This isn't the same colour as your eyes but compliments your natural shade and it will make your eyes really pop.

5   **A statement lip**
There is a bold lip shade out there for everyone. See page 42 if you're not yet convinced.

6   **A little bit of shimmer for your eyes**
It's all about bringing light. And no, you are never too old for some subtle eye shimmer, it's just about where you place it.

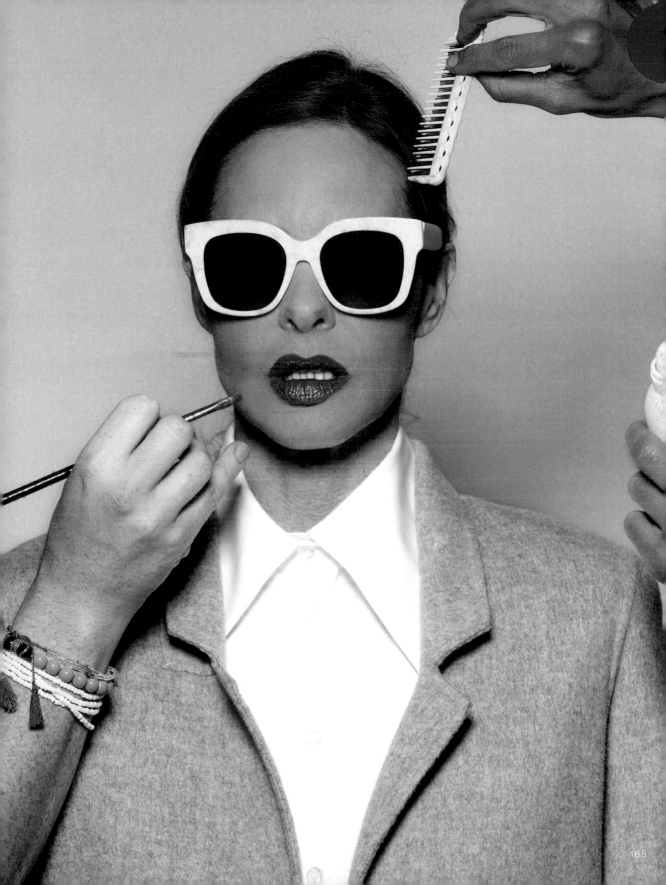

All about the base...

The very first thing I want to say here is: own the colour of your skin. Whatever your natural skin colour is, it is beautiful. You do not need to try to change it.

Take it from someone who spent much of her teens caked in fake tan mousse in an attempt to hide her acne. Not a good idea.

Trying to alter your skin tone - with fake tan, bronzer or a base the wrong shade - will put that essential relationship between your skin, hair and eyes out of whack. You'll likely have a slight line around your hairline where the skin is a different tone. It will also dull your face.

What you choose will also depend on whether your skin tends towards oily or dry. Those with oily skin will probably prefer not to add more shine with a heavier weight product. Those with dry skin will want to lean towards adding back some glow.

In order of weight, from low to high, these are products we can use as a base:

A skin perfector is not much more than a light moisturiser with a small amount of pigment.

A tinted serum contains active ingredients as well as giving you some light coverage. It provides another opportunity to address a skin concern in addition to your skincare products.

Tinted moisturisers offer some level of hydration alongside coverage, though not usually much in the way of actives.

Sheer coverage foundation is the lightest kind of foundation.

Radiant coverage foundation is formulated to give a very dewy look and is hydrating.

Satin coverage foundation sits in the middle of radiant and matt, in terms of how much glow it brings to your complexion.

Matt coverage foundation lacks luminosity and the product tends to feels thicker. This is the least light reflecting foundation that will give most coverage.

It's important to say that you don't have to wear any base at all. You might just dab on a bit of concealer and be good to go. Or you might wear a light base when your face is feeling a bit tired.

Less is more here. If you are someone who is used to wearing a heavy foundation then it can feel exposing to wean yourself off but I promise that a lighter base with a focus on the natural tones and light in your skin will feel more comfortable and more freeing. Thick foundations can flatten the face and take away character.

How to apply your base

Stage 1: Start by applying your base where you most need it. For the majority of us, this will be in the middle of our face, around our nose. Don't cover up your best skin first or you'll end up putting on twice as much as you actually need.

Stage 2: Blend it outwards from there. The aim is to give yourself light coverage using only as much base as you need to even out your skin tone. Blending is so important for this and will also help it to sink into your skin rather than just sit there. Which gives you a good canvas for whatever you want to add next.

Note: You might find that all you need is a small amount of coverage around your nose and chin, blended well over the top of a tinted serum that you have first put on all over.

Note: Go easy under the eye – particularly if you are applying a heavier product and you have reached that stage on the path of life where the skin there has become slightly crepe-y. Under-eye concealer is the best thing for the job here.

Getting the right colour base and concealer for your skin is so important. And of course this may change slightly or a lot, depending on whether it's summer or winter, just as your skincare concerns change with the season. There are many ways to buy makeup online and get a colour that's right for you. If you are shade matched in a store, always go outside to look at it in daylight and decide for yourself if it's right before you buy it.

Concealer

Under the eye:

The skin under your eye is more delicate and has fewer oil glands. You may also have more fine lines and some puffiness here. So we are looking for something with a lighter, cream consistency that will go on easily and move with our skin. Under-eye concealers described as 'buildable' can be layered to give more coverage on days when you feel you need it.

Avoid making under the eye much lighter. Years ago, when YSL's Touche Éclat first came on the market and pens were all the rage, we were encouraged to go much lighter with our under-eye concealer as a way of counteracting dark circles. I really don't think this panda eye approach helps; it just means the whole face doesn't come together. If you have particularly dark circles, you can try a slightly lighter concealer in the corners closest to your nose. Otherwise, your concealer should be the same colour as your foundation and the same colour as your face.

To cover spots, redness, hyperpigmentation:

Elsewhere on your face, a thicker concealer that will stay in one place will be more effective. If you are covering up an angry spot then you will need something packed with pigment and robust.

But concealer isn't just about hiding things we don't like. Some lighter concealers can do much of the work of making our complexion even. Some of us may even find that we need very little base, or can switch to something lighter, if we get our concealer right.

Always blend. Never let it just sit on top of your skin.

Bronzer

If you have a minimalist approach to makeup you may assume bronzer is not worth the faff. Or if you have a deep or pale complexion, you tried a one-size-fits-all version in the past and felt it didn't look right on your skin, you might be reluctant to go back there.

There is a big difference between a natural looking cream bronzer that comes in different shades and the orangey, shimmery powers you might be thinking of when you hear the word 'bronzer'.

What a good bronzer is bringing to the party is a touch of sun-kissed healthy glow that adds depth with just a swipe without being noticeable in itself. It is a hardworking product that takes mere seconds to apply. To find the right one, consider the colour you naturally tan, if you do. You want something that is a couple of shades darker than your foundation. Crucially, avoid anything with lots of shimmer and instead go for a subtle luminosity.

Bronzer goes on the 'high points' of your face, where you would naturally catch the sun. With a small amount on your finger, start from your temple and draw a C shape that ends in line with the corner of your eye. Then another from there across the top of your cheek bones - like a number three on each side of your face. Add a further touch to your nose and the middle of your chin and blend with a brush or clean fingers.

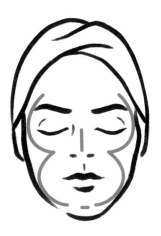

Blusher

Blusher brings an immediate flush of life like nothing else can. They key is to use just enough in the right places.

There are other places than our cheeks to place blusher. Most of us will naturally flush a little on our foreheads and on our nose too, so a light swipe in these places adds to that 'just been for a brisk walk' rosiness.

There are different types of blusher available:

Cream blushers are by far my favourite. They are easy and quick to apply with fingers or a brush and sit more naturally on the skin. They also wear better as you go about your day.

Liquid blusher give a wash of colour, a bit like a stain. They tend to dry quickly, so you need to apply them with a brush or your fingers. There's not much margin for error here and you only need a small amount.

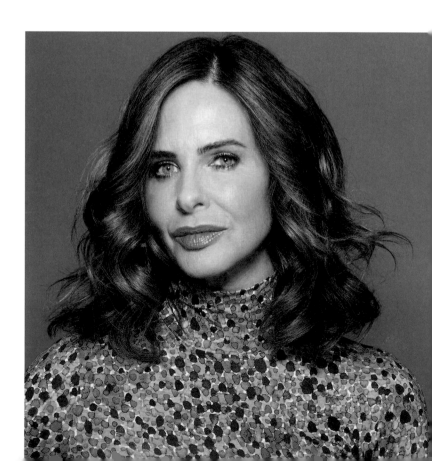

Powder blushers also require a brush. They can be matt or have a slight shimmer. They are fairly easy to apply and blend but as they are fine they don't always stay where they are put. They can disappear into your base and need reapplication later in the day or cling to and highlight areas of dryness. They can also be a bit flat.

If you have redness in your skin that you tone down with concealer or base, then you might not want to add it back with blusher. But bringing in this natural flush will be flattering so long as you put the blusher in the right place and choose a shade that's right for you. While we do want our base to create a sense of evenness, we also want to honour our natural tones so as not to flatten our features.

Keep your lip the same tone as your blusher, so there is a flow. For your face shape, see page 18.

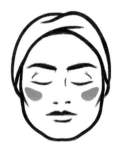

Square

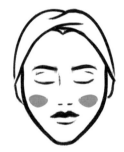

Heart

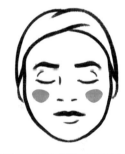

Round

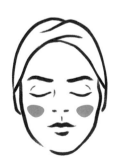

Oval

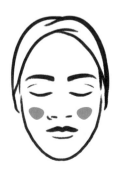

Long Oval

If you have a narrow face then apply blusher to the front, on the apples of your cheeks. Whereas if your face is broader you can bring it out further to the sides. If you feel it's bringing your face shape down then you have applied it too low - it should give a lift.

Highlighter

While bronzer usually deepens your skin tone for a just-been-on-holiday look, a highlighter is the same colour as your skin and is all about bringing light and luminosity. Again, avoid anything too glittery. You are going for dewy radiance rather than Disney princess. And cream based will feel more subtle than powder.

If you are new to highlighter, start with that C shape again, but this time from your temple, around your eye and across the top of your cheekbone. If there is a clash with your blusher, you are going too low with one or too high with the other. And blend to get a soft-focus effect, avoiding a 'stripe' moment.

How to elevate

Happy with the effect? You can also try a small amount immediately above and below the eyebrow for a subtle lift, and the lightest touch down the centre of the nose and in the cupids bow. Don't go overboard as you might start to look oily. Focus on the areas where the light naturally hits your face (go and stand next to a window if you aren't sure) and experiment until you have achieved a subtle but radiant glow.

Step 1

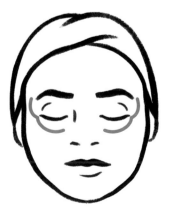

Step 2

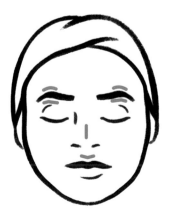

The eyes

The focus of our face – our most important feature and the one that we really want to pop.

When we put on a print that doesn't quite work because it's wearing us, we can tell because our eyes get lost. This is where we almost always want to pull focus.

Our eyes change as we go down the path of life – or rather, the shape and texture of the skin around them does. So it's important to have an awareness of what's best for the woman you are today. There is no reason why you can't wear a colour on your lid at any stage of life, it's just about doing it in a way that works for you.

Makeup for hooded eyes

A hooded eye, where the skin below the brow hangs over the lid, is by far the most common eye shape. Many of us are born with them or our eyes head that way with age. There's nothing wrong with this. These are some of the ways to make them look open and lifted.

- If you have slightly oily eyelids, you probably find that oil builds up in the crease, so start with a mattifying primer, giving your eye shade something to grab onto.

- Choose a lighter shade for the inner corner of the eyelid and a darker shade on the outside, to avoid heaviness. Or if you are using one colour, don't build it on the inside.

- Take the colour quite high under your brow bone, to alter the sense of where the crease is, blending so it's not harsh.

- At the outer corner of the eye, make sure the colour is lifted up towards your brow, rather than creeping down, where it will drag your eye down. Use a ring finger to blend the towards the temple.

- If you want to, you can add a sliver of highlighter just under the middle of the brow.

Eyeliner

Eyeliner can be many things. It can be rock chic cool, with a smudged and sexy smokey eye; it can be creative strokes and bright colours to show individuality; a French flick for sophistication, or, it can be the thing that really ages you.

Let us start with that last one. If you are fifty or above, the problem with a hard eyeliner is that it can close up the eye and make it look smaller, when we are trying to open up the eye, in order to make us look more energised and awake.

If you are in your thirties or forties and you feel that a swipe of liquid eyeliner with a flick is still very much your look and you're not ready to part with it then that's absolutely fine. Personality is an important part of the way we choose to do our makeup. But if your eyes have become hooded over time, this might be the moment you need to let go and I would ask, have you thought about experimenting with something softer? If you use a kohl eyeliner, how about blending it for a subtler look? It could be the time to challenge ourselves.

I sometimes use a metallic crayon around my inner eye to bring some light.

Whenever I use an eyeliner, I put a touch of concealer under my eyes and sweep it up towards the outer corners of my eyebrows to ensure that nothing is dragging my face or eyes down.

Love the skin you are in

Open your eyes

Before

After

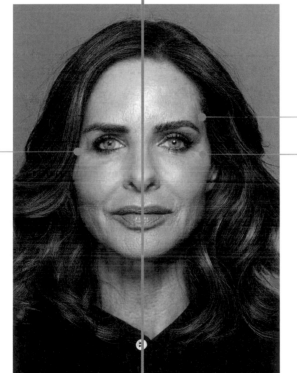

I will brush my eyebrows upwards to give impact and open up the eyes.

A hard black liner will drag the eye down and make it look smaller.

In a very soft way, I use black liner blended along my lashline to make my lashes appear more dense, rather than to have the appearance of a line. This will open the eyes and make your look more alert and bright.

Eyelashes

Let's go back to basics for a moment, as it's always good to make sure we aren't neglecting the simple things.

- Don't neglect those very fine hairs on the inside of the eye. Make sure they get a swipe of mascara too.

- Get product into the lash roots to give volume. Twizzle the brush at the root before drawing it through the lashes.

- Mascara dries quickly, so work on one eye at a time.

- For the final flourish, make sure any excess mascara is removed from the brush and gently touch the lower lashes.

- Before the mascara dries, run through with an eyelash comb to separate out the lashes and remove any clumps.

Mascara is a product with a shorter shelf life. If you find it's thicker and clumpier, it is time for a new one. If it starts to smell, it has gone off. As you pump it, you release oxygen into the formulation and it will dry out faster, so do avoid doing this.

Lash serums

Good lash serums do work. Note that they can make your eyelashes grow at different angles and they may irritate if you have very sensitive eyes. Do note, some contain dye that can slightly transfer and make it look like you have dark circles. Do your research and find one that really works.

Eyelash extensions

Eyelashes done by an experienced professional who takes responsibility for your eyelash health is an easy way to always look great. You should never have more than one hair extension on one of your natural lashes, and generally no longer than 2mm longer than your natural lash length. There are different types and a good technician will look at your eye socket shape to decide yours.

Brows

Eyebrows frame the face. Even as our face softens, our brows still bring structure. Small changes here can make a big difference.

If you fell victim to the overplucking trend of the nineties and early noughties, you might not have as much eyebrow as you would like. Or you might be used to the thinner shape you have and be wary about changing it.

There are two things to consider. If you have brows that are thicker nearer your nose and slim at the outer edges, it can contribute to a 'furrowed brow' effect. You may find a more even width will balance this out, and make you notice emerging frown lines less.

The other thing is the curve of your brow. Some women look great with a high arch but if the outside edge goes into too much of a downward curve it can pull your whole eyeshape down. If you also have undereye shadow, this will create an odd circle around your eye. Often, a straighter line, lowering the arch, gives a lifted effect.

The only note of caution here is that you don't want your brows to be so heavy – in terms of size and colour – that they are the first thing someone notices when they look at your face. Brows provide architecture but the focus should always be the eyes themselves.

Get an eyebrow pencil and have a play in the mirror. You can draw on heavy, oversize brows if you want, just to get a feel for changes to brow shape have an effect on how we see the face. Then, if you feel like you need some advice or a fresh perspective, go and see a brow expert (remember to take the drawn-on eyebrows off first).

Brow gel

This feels a bit like mascara for your brows, not least because the wand is like a smaller version of a 'spoolie' that you use to apply mascara. It is very easy to use, adds definition, tames unruly brows and helps covers sparse areas. The key is to first go against the direction that the hair grows in, then back the other way to neaten, ensuring the product coats both sides.

A neutral lip

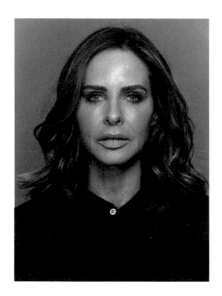

A washed out neutral lip

If you choose just one shade too light, it will wash out your whole complexion and make your face look flat and lifeless.

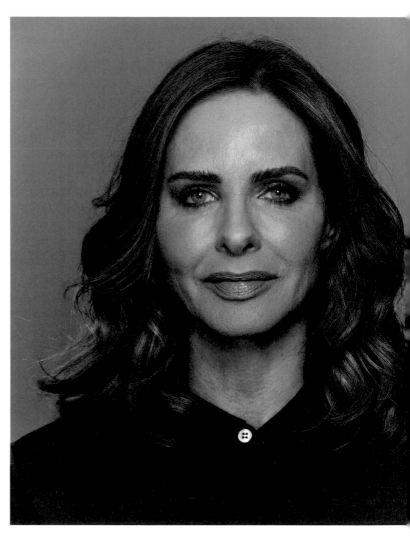

A tonal neutral lip

Instead, use a lip tone that is one shade darker than your lips. This will bring life to your whole face and will bring your makeup look together.

A red lip

I am not wearing an
eyeshadow that clashes with
the lip. Instead I have used
a shade that helps to frame
the socket and create depth.
I have applied lots of mascara
to help to frame the eye and
add balance to the face.

If you aren't sure what blusher
shade to use, you can cheat by
using a tiny bit of the lipstick
colour. Lightly apply this to the
cheeks and you will ensure you
have the right tone.

A red lip always makes me feel
confident. As with everything,
it largely comes down to
whether you are cool or warm
toned (see page 28). As a
general underlying rule, when
we are talking about red lips,
shades with a blue undertone
or that skew pinky are best for
cools and those with a orange
base are best for warms. Look
to pages 40–45 for possible lip,
cheek and eye combinations.

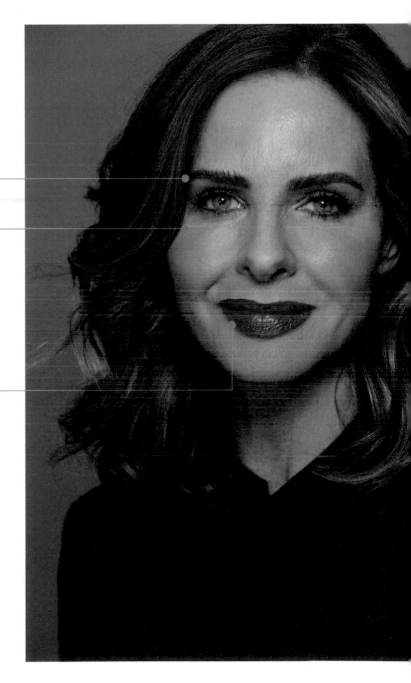

Nighttime glamour

To me nighttime glamour is when I present a face that has no memory of the day that might have made me tired. I look in the mirror and I feel sexy and confident. The question is, how do I get there?

1   **Prep is key.** Take off your makeup from the day, complete your skincare routine again and give your face a massage. You will wake up your skin and make it ready for feeling glamorous.

2   **Get the glow.** The ultimate glamorous finish is glowy skin. To get this subtle glow from within your skin, you put your highlighter on before your base. I do this with contour too, and everything just looks softer.

3   **It's all about the eyes.** This is not about a lip. Start with the lighter shade and add a wash across your eyelid up into the socket and slightly over. Using a small, flat brush, line underneath your lower lash line and across your upper lash line from about halfway, meeting in the outer corner of your eye. I will add in an extra bit of shimmer on the inside of my top and bottom lashline to give that inner sparkle to my eyes.

4   **Lips should be kissable.** They are secondary, but they should absolutely not be neglected. Opt for a neutral shade, one shade deeper than your natural lip colour. It could be in matt to define the shape, and then use a product with a little bit of sheen and put it in the middle of your lip. Add a touch of this to your blusher for the extra shimmer.

No one-size-fits-all in makeup

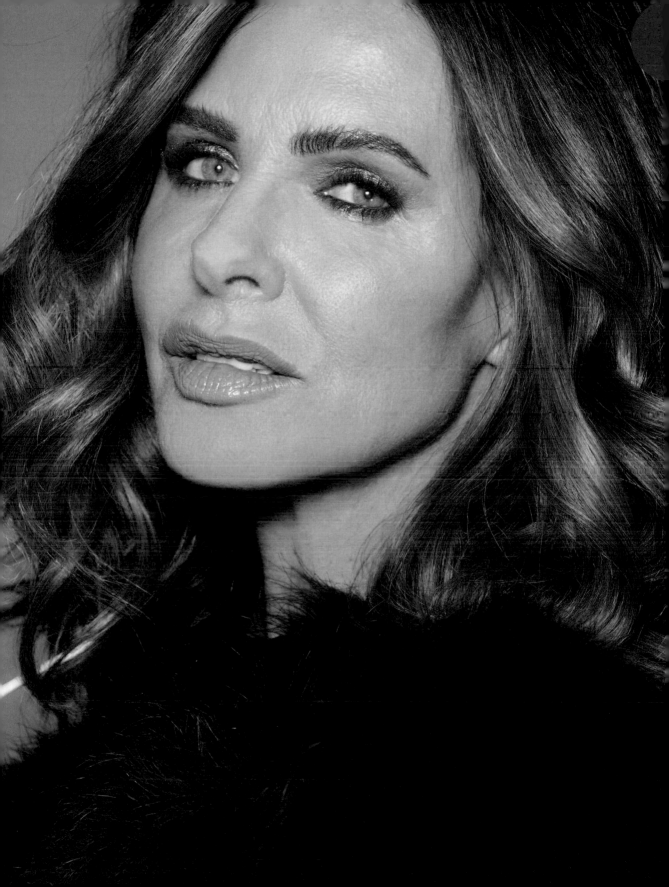

ASK YOURSELF

1   Have you worn the same products for over 10 years?

2   Are you someone who has never worn makeup and don't know where to start?

3   When you do your makeup, how much do you see the texture on your face (i.e. the powders)?

4   Have you changed your go-to lip colour in the last decade?

5   Does your foundation match your skin tone?

CHALLENGE YOURSELF

1   Our faces change as we age, so we do need to change the things we use and how we apply them. Every 10 years, look through what you have in your drawer, look at the elements of your face that have changed and refresh your products to ensure that you always look your best.

2   If you haven't really worn makeup before, give yourself a gentle introduction. Try a BB cream to see how your skin can glow, or invest in a blusher to lift the colour that might be fading on your face. Or you could just try one product that you can use on your lip, cheek and eyes and experiment with it. Just be sure to stick to the colours that suit you (see page 15).

3   It might be time to step away from a powder base and try using cream alternatives. Even if that means using your lipstick as a blusher. Try this the next time you are putting on your makeup and see how the cream sits as part of your skin rather than on top of it.

4   Our lip colour changes over time too. What suited us 10 years ago, may now be too harsh. If you love the colour, look to see if you might be able to get it in a shade that now suits you. I always recommend selecting a neutral that is one shade darker than your skin tone to add a little contrast.

5   It is vital to pick the right shade of foundation for your skin. Love the skin you are in and don't try to hide it, you should be enhancing it. As fine lines start to appear, foundations that may have previously worked may not do any longer. The foundation may start to gather, and make any lines more prominent. If you are used to wearing a lot of makeup, this is a time to consider selecting a lighter product and applying it more lightly too.

FEAR
LESS

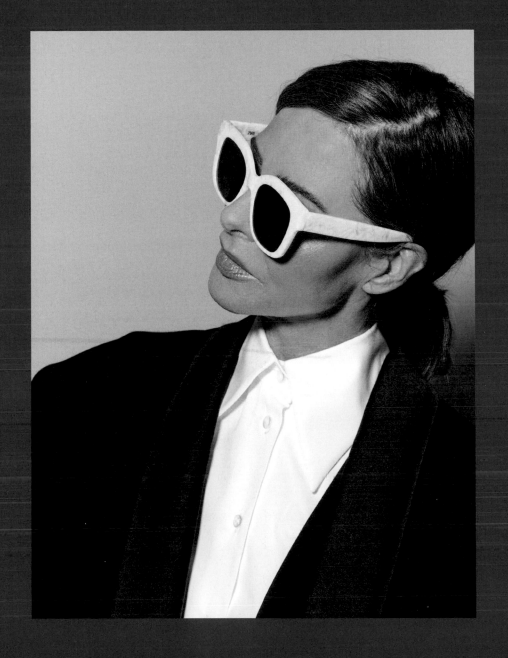

STYLE

COLOUR
BRINGS

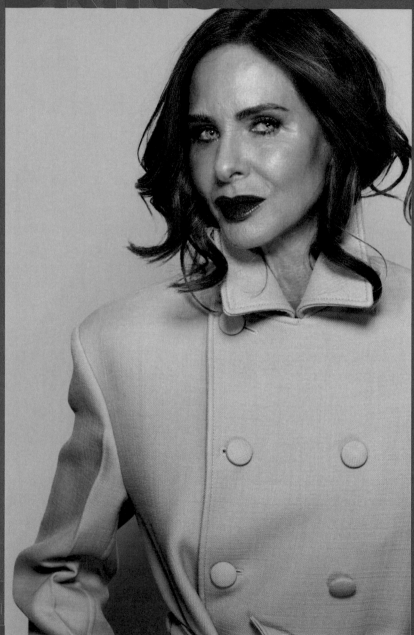

LIFE

Why care about what to wear?

What you choose to put on in the morning is about so much more than the clothes themselves. What we wear has the power to make us feel more confident, energised and joyful.

It can help us to fully become the women we want to be and help you get there quicker. But it is also very emotional and sometimes can make us put up barriers that stop us from challenging ourselves to project who we really are. This is what I want this book to do for you - challenge you.

I feel so much more confident now than I did in my twenties. There are still days when I wake up and feel less sure of myself. Perhaps I'm going into a work situation when I have to make an impression. On these days, I will wear something that makes me totally present in the room. This gives me an opening to find my voice, catch up with myself and ease into confidence. I used to lay out twenty outfits on the bed, thinking, 'Who am I today?' Now, instead, I think, 'Which part of me do I want to channel? What do I want to bring into the room today?'

Perhaps you are moving into a new stage in your life and you don't yet know how to inhabit it. Or you might be feeling a little lost and unsure about what suits you. This is when we need to take control and one way is to be intentional about how we dress. I've made over thousands of women around the world and I have seen again and again the confidence that comes from leaning into who we want to be and wearing the clothes that illustrate that person.

What we wear has the power to make us feel fearless

FEEL INSPIRED

In this part, I want to inspire you to reflect on how you dress and to look at it differently.

Just as I would if we met in person, I'm going to ask you to consider your style journey so far.

It is about so much more than clothes.

When you are fearless in how you dress you'll be amazed by the responses you'll get from people in your life and how utterly transformed you will feel.

We carry associations and baggage regarding what we wear, even without consciously realising it. Sometimes they simply form our personal preferences but they can also be emotional roadblocks, which get in the way of dressing as the women we want to the world to see.

In this part, I will guide you to become confident in your colour choices and teach you how to elevate any outfit and reinvigorate old clothes. If you understand how you dress now, you can take the next new challenge of presenting yourself with joy and without fear.

What is your style?

When I first meet a woman I can always interpret an element of who she is by how she presents herself and what she wears.

There are many reasons why we choose certain clothes other than taste or conscious preference. I wonder what has taken you to where you are now?

Before you start

Let's take a step back and ask some questions about what lies behind your style choices. Knowing this and owning it is the key when you decide to make a change. If something is holding you back then let's find out what it is so we can clear the way to where you want to get to.

There are some common beliefs and insecurities that influence what we choose to wear that I see often.

How do you see yourself?

Time and time again I have come across women who hide the most extreme aspect of their individuality in order to conform to how they think the world should see them. So, I'm going to ask you now, where do you give yourself oxygen? Where do you suffocate your style? I know that the fear of judgement can sometimes be overwhelming.

Over the next few pages, I've highlighted five aspects of dressing that will help you understand how you communicate with your body on an emotional level. These definitely do not cover all styles of dressing, they are just core elements to look at.

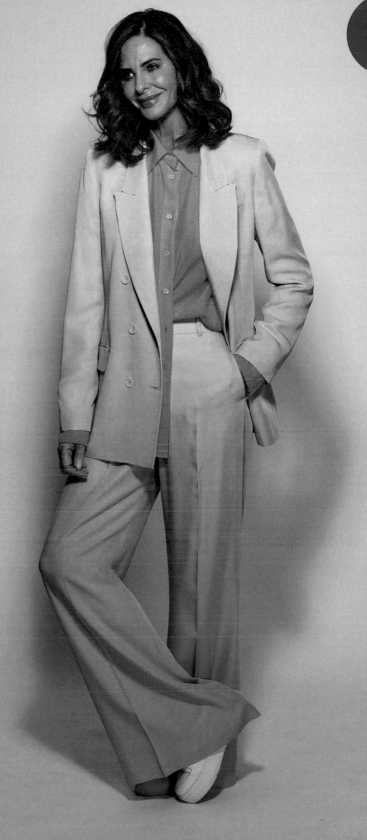

Your style habits

We use our clothes to project different aspects of our personality.

You might be like me and use a few of these elements, depending on the day and how you are feeling. The question I want you to ask yourself is: do you rely on any of these too often? By doing so, do you hide who you really are from the world? We can choose to let our body dictate how we dress, or we can choose how we want to see our body and dress to complement it. If you wear the same look every day of the week, it is time to try something new one day a week so that you can slowly but surely build your confidence and positive relationship with your body.

The maxi-dresser

Sometimes volume is wonderfully stylish, but equally it can be used as a way to hide our emotional relationship with our body. We can choose to dress this way in order to make ourselves feel more comfortable. The best way to do this look is to not use it as a way to disguise the elements of yourself you may not like. We are generally our own harshest critics. You need to learn to show more of yourself and build your courage. Instead of using voluminous items with no shape, try the concept of layering instead (see page 272).

The intellectual

I have met many women who say how they dress isn't important to them, or they have no interest in fashion. Many have jobs that require a uniform. But you should always consider how you are presenting yourself. Give yourself permission to see clothing as an extension of your personality, a way to show your vulnerability. It is worth experimenting (try the examples on page 290) and it might even become an enjoyable passion ...

The warm and cosy

In a post-pandemic world, warm and cosy has become a far bigger way of dressing, as comfort is now key. When we get used to dressing one way for a long time, it can be a real challenge to up the ante. There is nothing wrong with looking like we are just back from the gym, but you are doing yourself a disservice if this is your everyday look. If you are most comfortable in sweatpants and a T-shirt, it is time for you to think about fantastic sports luxe. With this as your base, you can then start to incorporate smarter elements, such as a T-shirt with a long silk skirt or a tailored jacket with sweat pants.

Loud but shy

This is an interesting oxymoron and it definitely applies to me sometimes. It can be fabulous to wear bright colours as they are so inviting to others, but it can conversely be used as a way to hide. On days I am feeling less confident, I will often reach for the wildest outfits to obscure how I feel. Instead, you want to wear clothes that make you feel present and bright. This is why wearing the right shades of a colour and their contrasting tones can really make a big difference to how you look and feel (see page 210), taking your fearless dressing to the next level.

The body-confident dresser

I want every one of you to become this person and to love and accept your body. You should always understand and appreciate your body, and, yes, you should show it off. This doesn't mean you have to have lots of flesh on show. It is about choosing clothing that shows off both your body and your personality. Your style of dressing may evolve as your body shape changes over the years, but I want your level of confidence to remain high.

ASK YOURSELF

1	Does your clothing celebrate your identity?
2	Do you view clothing as a way to hide?
3	Do you sometimes feel bored with the way you dress?
4	Does how you dress bring you joy?
5	How often do people comment on your outfit or ask you where it is from?

CHALLENGE YOURSELF

1	Look at your wardobe and ask yourself whether you duplicate the same style of item. Challenge yourself to stop buying repeats for a year.
2	If you wear the same style every day, challenge yourself to try something new one day a week. In month two do this two days a week, month three try three days and so on. Elevate your style by trying out some different types of dressing (see page 290).
3	How we think we are seen and how we are actually seen can be completely different. We don't need to hide. If someone gives you a compliment, write it down and refer back to it when you need to feel fearless. Acknowledge that people notice when we make an effort with how we present ourselves.

Who do you think you are?

The temptation is to fall back on old favourites that feel safe but don't challenge us to ask - who do we really want to be?

The more we have a sense of ourselves, the less we need in our wardrobe to distract us. We want to get to a place where we open those doors and see a rail of clothes that work for who we are, that we know how to style, and that make us feel confident and present when we put them on. When we ditch the things that don't live up to these standards and are left with the things that do we discover a fabulous ease of dressing. For some of us, it will be more of a journey to get to that point than for others, but for everyone, the process starts with letting go of the old you.

Most of us tend to wear 20% of our wardrobe 80% of the time.

It is in the details: necklines

Here's where being intentional about detail really pays off. A flattering neckline can elevate an outfit and turn it into something special. Knowing what works particularly well for you will give you even more confidence when you shop or put an outfit together.

I am asked a lot about necklines, so here I have included some of the best and worst for you. I wouldn't normally use that language, but here I will, as the suitability of a neckline will change with age. I used to focus the most on how boobs look, but now I find necklines have the most impact and we will feel fearless when we get it right.

Here is what to take into account:

The size of your boobs

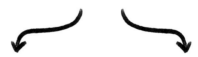

The width of your shoulders

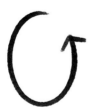

The shape of your face

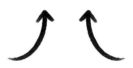

The length of your neck

Here are some general principles that I use when I'm styling myself and other women. I want to challenge you to go through your wardrobe and pull out examples of different necklines and decide which is the best for you and why.

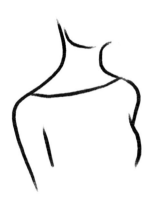

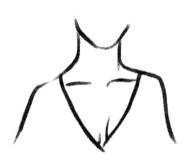

Boat

A high boat neck, especially in a horizontal stripe, is great to broaden out narrow shoulders and will make those with wider hips look more in proportion.

Deep V

Anyone can wear this style. It is good for narrow shoulders and for anyone with larger boobs as it breaks up the fabric with some skin. If the skin on your neck or chest has changed, move away from this style as you move along the path of life.

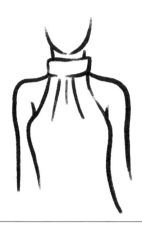

Halter

A halter neck is a great way for all of us to feel sexy and fearless. It is especially good for those with smaller boobs and broad shoulders, as it pulls colour near the face, making it the focus, and will emphasise the great shape of the shoulders.

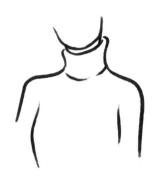

Polo Neck

If you have big boobs, wear this style with a jacket or with a long necklace to break up the expanse of fabric. A cowl neck over the age of fifty is difficult to wear as it will not bring any structure to your neck and it can therefore age you.

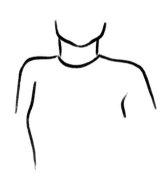

Round

A round neck is a style that everyone can wear as it is flattering and adds structure around the face. It is ageless. If you have bigger boobs, you might want to wear a jacket to break the line and lift the look.

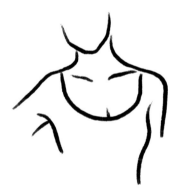

Scoop

The only neckline that is very hard for most women is a wide scoop neck, like a leotard. You should avoid it if you don't have boobs and your top half is a little bony.

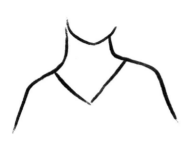

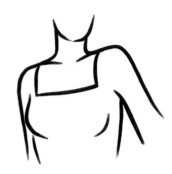

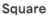

Shallow V

A shallow V will elongate the neck and is often flattering on those with round or heart-shaped faces.

Square

A square neck or bustier style neckline is a very strong look for any size and shape. If you have broad shoulders, this is a great choice as the neckline goes straight across.

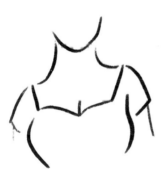

Sweetheart

If you have both boobs and hips, a gentle sweetheart neckline is the best choice as the flow of the style will emphasise your shape.

The length of a sleeve

I love a statement sleeve. I truly think there's a style for everyone, whether it's a dramatic leg-of-mutton, batwing or something more subtle:

A short sleeve

This is great for broadening out and bringing attention to the shoulder area. It is less good for those who would rather draw attention away from larger boobs as the sleeve finishes in line with the breast, so instead opt for elbow length.

An elbow length sleeve

Brings the attention to the waist. Perfect for those with an hourglass figure.

A three-quarter length sleeve

This is an elegant way to show a small amount of skin and is useful for balancing out volume and layering. This is great if you have a petite frame, though if you have very long arms, it will serve to make them look longer.

A bracelet sleeve

I always think this looks particularly good on petite women. If you have longer arms use bracelets to fill in the gap.

A full length sleeve (to back of hand)

A desirable length for the long of arm. It's also chic and will appeal to those whose style tends towards the classic.

Strike a pose

We spend so much time at desks or looking at screens that thinking about how we sit and stand is crucial.

Post-menopausal osteoporosis causes some of us to lose inches of height and become more rounded in the shoulder. But being aware of our posture is something we should all be doing, even if you're reading this and you're in your twenties. If you're a sloucher – and I definitely am, like lots of taller women – you need to be particularly aware of your posture (*did you just sit up straight when reading this?!*).

Good posture has an impact psychologically and aesthetically. Hunching over diminishes us. If you sit and stand up straight you will feel more confident and less tired. You will have more presence in the room. Engaging your core and pushing your shoulders back opens you up and allows you to breathe better, so you get more oxygen into your body. I do Pilates and I recognise how the work I do on my core helps me have a healthier back and better posture. If it is an issue for you, consider trying The Alexander Technique.

We can also choose clothes that accentuate our shape and give us back the sharper lines our body can lose as we age. If you have straight, broad shoulders wear drop shoulder coats and jackets (where the shoulder seam sits on your arm, below the natural line of your shoulder).

A well-cut jacket can work wonders for accentuating straight shoulders and good posture. And if you feel you have good posture, you are more likely to sit up straight.

Shoulder pads will always remind some of us of 1980's power dressing, but a well-placed pad can do so much for the drape of a top or jacket. I have a Zara T-shirt with a slim shoulder pad and it adds so much definition. You can also buy silicone ones online. Creating a straight line and adding a slight width to your shoulders with pads or tailoring will slim your waist and balance a large bust.

For those who are petite ...

I am always asked by petite ladies, 'But how can I wear that?' ... I believe that any woman can wear any style, it just depends on the proportions of an outfit.

Volume dressing

To avoid being swamped, don't hide your natural shape. Three-quarter or half-length sleeves will draw attention to your waist.

Waistline

This is where you can add in proportionality. I use a belt to lower the waist, but if you are petite you can use a belt to lift the waist.

Wide-legged trousers

Should not be discounted. Wearing a stacked trainer or wedge with a wide-leg trouser will help you to achieve flow in your outfit.

Layering

Everyone can layer. It is just about hitting the key layering points (see page 272).

Where to shop

Besides petite ranges, if you want fantastic tailoring consider the boys department. If the brand is sophisticated and also does adult clothing, you can also try certain girls departments.

Shoes

Go for thinner straps. Ankle straps may make you look shorter.

... and those who are tall

Being 5ft 10in, I sit in the category of a taller woman. Here are a few tips I use.

Sleeves

Often, especially on the high street, the sleeves will be cut too short for me. They make me feel like an orangutan. If it is in a jacket then I can pull the cuff of a jumper or top through, bringing more texture and colour. Alternatively, chunky cuff bracelets can fill the gap around my wrist caused by a too-short sleeve length. But I have now stopped buying jackets that are too short in the arm, as I know ultimately I will wear them much less.

Wearing heels

If you are someone with very slim legs you might prefer to avoid chunky-soled or block-heel shoes. Never feel you can't wear heels, no matter your height. Never apologise for being a tall woman ...

Any woman can wear any style

Check your specs

In terms of eyewear, finding the right shape for you often requires some experimentation. Take a friend with you when you go to try on glasses and don't forget to put on some makeup as you will be looking at your face quite close up - if you feel you look tired you are far more likely to give up and go home. Take advice from the people who work in the store but ultimately you know your style, your personality and the colours you wear most, so don't be talked into something you don't feel is right.

Where does the frame finish?

You don't want the frames to sit outside your temple. If you have a narrow face you will find this is even more important. Does the shape/dimensions of the glasses drag down your face?

This is a consideration for everyone, but if you have an oval face without very prominent cheekbones you will find that a curve lower down on your face will pull everything down.

Do the glasses wear you?

Just like with a bold print, you don't want your face to get lost behind your statement glasses. Take a step back from the mirror - are the glasses the first thing you see?

Can I wear statement jewellery?

Wearing glasses can be hard with statement earrings, as they will fight for attention and may make your face feel overcrowded. The best way to make it all work together is, as ever, to make sure there's a certain flow. If the colour of the glasses - particularly the arm - match your earrings and the shapes don't fight then there will be a continuity. You might prefer to keep any earrings subtle and focus on choosing glasses that make you feel cool.

For your face shape

Refer to page 18 to work out your face shape and discover the best shape and styles that will suit you.

Square

Try a style with soft edges. Round or aviator frames can look great; also consider cat-eye or butterfly-shaped frames.

Heart

Your best glasses will balance out the ratio between your brows and your chin – an aviator style or round shape frame – as they won't emphasise the wide or narrow areas.

Round

Square, rectangular or more unusual frame shapes are great for bringing structure. Frames that are wider at the top, like a butterfly shape, will draw the eye in and give balance.

Oval

You have lots of options. Square glasses will look more striking and emphasise your facial contours, while round glasses will have a softer effect.

Long Oval

These tend to suit a range of styles, though it can be best to avoid narrow frames as these can make your face appear longer.

Triangle

You'll look best in frames with a density to the browline and go as wide or wider than your jaw, like a cat-eye or aviator. A rounded, narrower bottom to the frame will soften your cheekbones.

Long Forehead

Those with a long forehead will look good in a frame that is tall and oversized. You want to find a frame that has a lifted browline bridge. An aviator style gives the illusion of shortening your face.

Short Forehead

If you have a short forehead, you want to avoid anything that goes above your browline.

Know your style and your personality

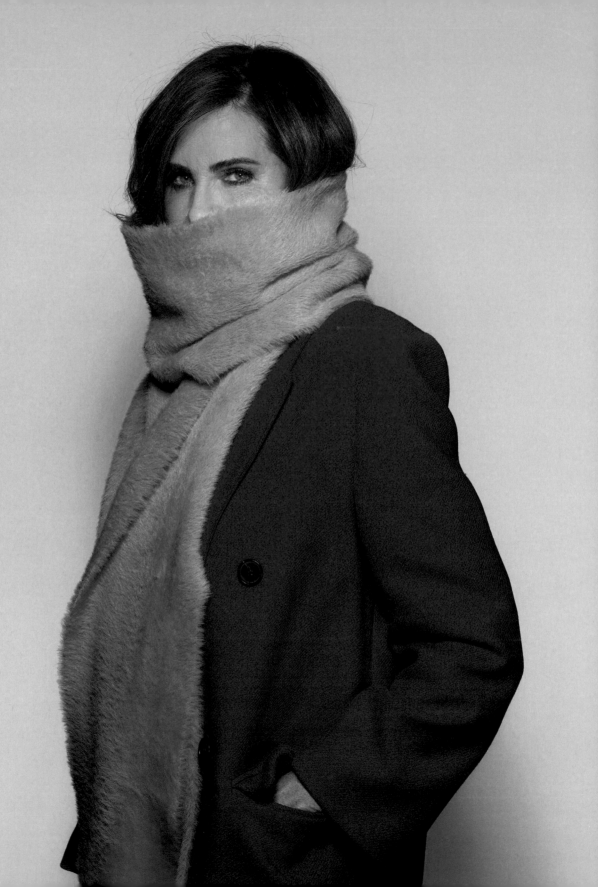

Colour me happy

I sometimes think I will have 'wear colour with colour' written on my gravestone. If you are not confident with colour there is a temptation to wear it with black as it can feel easier and safer. But not only does black drain the life from colour, wearing a colour on your top half and black on your bottom half will cut you off across the middle, so you won't get flow through an outfit.

Most importantly, there is so much fun to be had from mixing different shades. Or going all out with one colour and wearing it top to toe. I really notice the difference in how I feel and how people respond to me when I am wearing strong colour.

When you embrace colour and colour, it gives you many more options with your existing wardrobe. Clothes that you love and yet have been languishing at the back of your cupboard are given a whole new lease of life when you get creative about what you wear them with.

Go and have a look at some prints you already own. That scarf you love – what shades are in it and how are they working together? What else do you own in those tones? If you were to remove every black item from your wardrobe, how much is left and how can you build an outfit from those pieces?

I am not saying no to wearing black. Black works amazingly with neutrals like white and grey, but this is about bringing colour into your life.

Here, I will take you through how the core colours can work for you. Also, do see the Identify Yourself section on page 13.

Wear colour with colour

Opposites attract

So, how do you decide what colours will work together for you? This is a question I am asked possibly more than any other. Wearing colour with colour can feel intimidating but it really is one of the most joyful things.

Colours that sit next to each other on the colour wheel create a more subtle look but it's those that sit opposite one another that give us a striking contrast and therefore the most exciting combinations. You don't have to go the full enchilada with an entire outfit of strong opposites if you're not ready for that – start with a hint here and there, in a bag or some jewellery or a scarf, and see where it takes you.

Now it gets a little more technical. To really nail those colour combinations we need to consider the depth of tone. Look at the strength of the colour and match the levels. We can describe tones as soft or bright, cool or warm, dirty or clean.

Whatever your level of comfort with colour, I would love you to get out some favourite clothes and accessories in contrasting colours. Use the wheel as inspiration to try out combinations. Don't worry about whether you would actually wear those things together yet – just play to start with.

Start with a hint and see where it takes you

Colour wheel

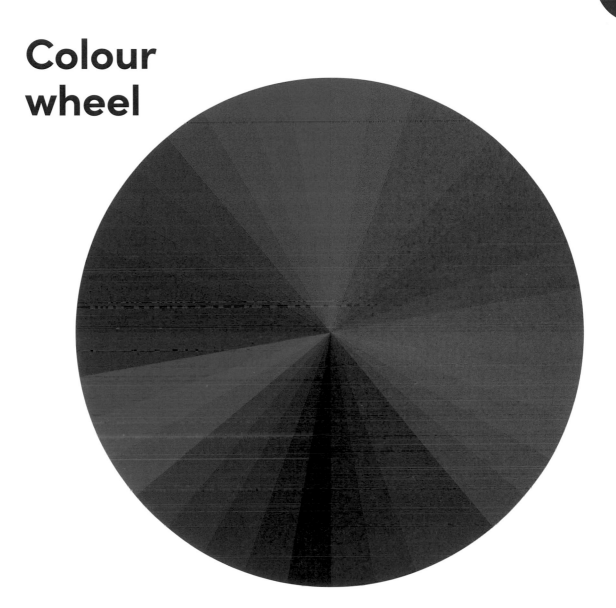

ASK YOURSELF

What do people say is your best shade and that you look good in?

What makes your heart sing?

What colours have you never thought to try before?

Which colours bring each other to life?

GREY

We might feel like grey stays in the background, or that it can be a brilliant accent for an electric shock of a bold colour, like bright magenta or acid yellow, but grey is also tremendously chic. Some of you might find grey reminds you of your school uniform, and you therefore have an uncomfortable relationship with it. But there are many shades of grey, and for the right skin tone it can be an amazing addition to your wardrobe.

- As all greys are cool, if you are cool or a cool/neutral, most tones will work for you.

- If you are a neutral, a very soft dove grey or a charcoal grey works well.

- If you're a warm/neutral or warm, you may need to think more about your makeup so the colour doesn't wash you out. Consider greys at the beige end of the scale in terms of their suitability.

Unlike navy, there are a few greys that won't work together. It plays nicely with most other colours too. Mixing different tones of grey is one of my favourite dress-down weekend looks, but then when you introduce some life and light - like a sequin or some silver, perhaps coupled with a smokey eye - you have the basis of a glamorous nighttime look. It gives the sophistication we might look to black for, but it's softer and often easier to wear.

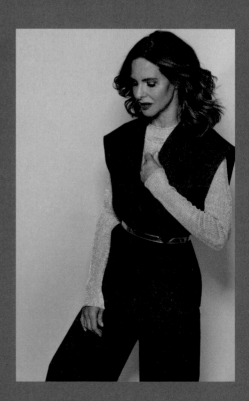

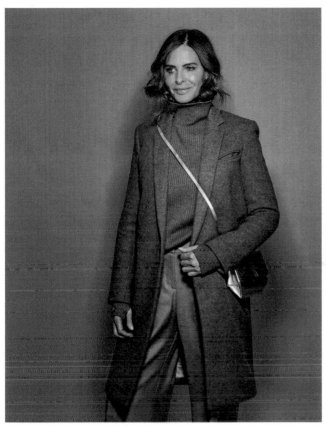

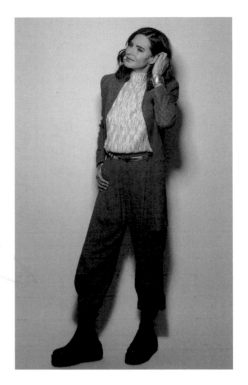

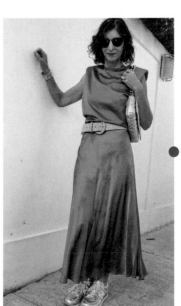

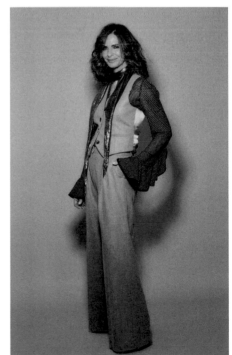

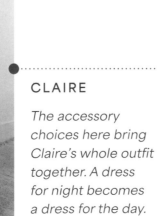

CLAIRE

The accessory choices here bring Claire's whole outfit together. A dress for night becomes a dress for the day.

NEUTRALS

Nothing beats the crisp coolness of white for bringing a classy but modern edge to proceedings. Of course, white might be broderie anglaise on holiday, but it is also a classic white shirt under a red suit or an elegant white coat. While black often shouts down other colours it comes into contact with, white and cream can elevate them. The first question to ask is, which is your white?

- If you are a cool or a cool/neutral, then true white is your good friend.

- Ecru is for neutral, for example if you have just a hint of red in your hair and cool grey or hazel eyes.

- Cream is warm and will work for you if are a warm or warm/neutral, with peachy, yellow or caramel tones to your skin.

You can absolutely mix the tones - whites get along well together - just wear your 'white' closest to your face. And all can be accessorised with either silver or gold, depending on what is best for your tones. A red lip is joyous with white but it's good to celebrate the crispness of the white by keeping our makeup clean and fresh.

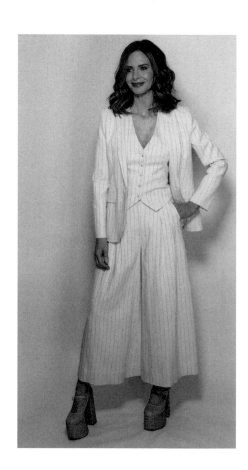

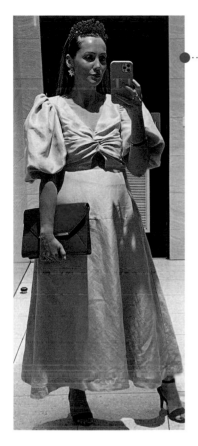

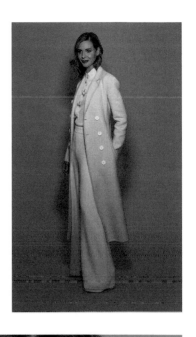

KATIE

I love the continued pop of colour on Katie's accessories that have been introduced to uplift this dress and add personality.

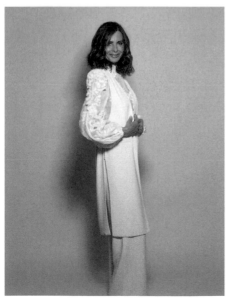

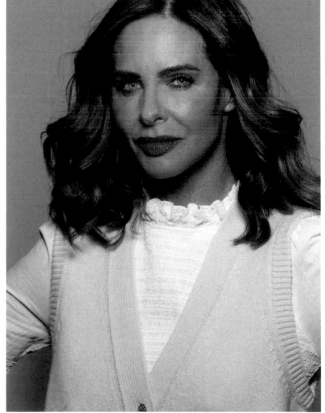

PINK FAMILY

Pink is often regarded as the most feminine of colours. The lighter shades evoke a sense of youth and innocence. It's never a threatening colour and even the brighter shades have a certain softness.

- If you are cool then you will want to go for the coolest, blue-based pinks. Pale rose and strong fushia pink are cool toned, while shocking or hot pink generally works. If you are a cool/neutral you may also suit a dirty raspberry shade.

- Dirty pink is often best for neutrals, into warm/neutral.

- Warm-toned people will suit dark raspberry.

Different shades of pink have lots of friends across the colour wheel. I love the femininity of a pastel pink contrasted with a bottle green and the exuberance of a bright pink and yellow combo. The only colour I avoid is blue - there is something dated about it.

As we go down the path of life and naturally lose definition in our features, we start to find that the extreme ends of our colour palette can become too harsh and wash us out. This is where thinking about shape becomes important too.

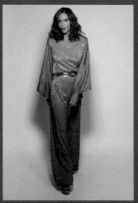 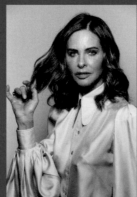 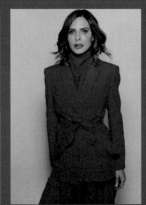

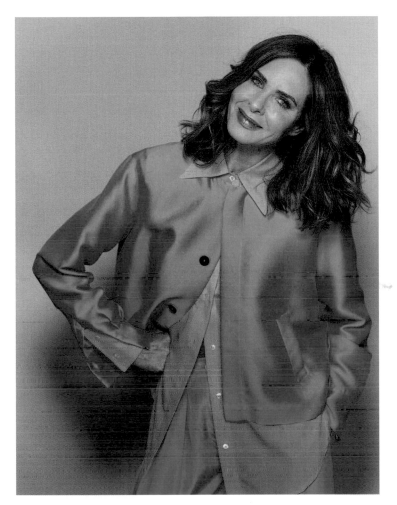

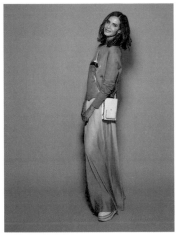

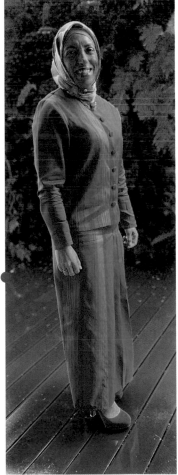

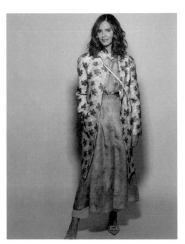

ANEEKAH

What an outfit. It is balanced and stylish and entirely confident! I love the peek of the complementary shoes too!

ORANGE FAMILY

Orange is such an uplifting and playful colour. It brings a youthful energy and vitality without severity. It also has a great relationship with pink and red and it's a lot of fun to play with different tones of these colours together, as unexpected combinations will pop up. Unlike blue or green, the spectrum of colours we consider to be orange is quite narrow - it really boils down to four main shades, plus neon.

- If you are cool, a strong, classic orange may work well for you. Apricot is a difficult colour - it is often best for cool/neutral blondes with peaches-and-cream complexions and if you're cooler (but not very cool) with dark-toned skin.

- If you are a neutral, salmon may be your shade.

- Rust is the warmest orange and it can be magnificent if you have red hair.

If you have a rosy complexion then you might be unsure about wearing orange as it brings out the redness of your skin. But if you love orange and if it works for your hair and your eye, consider using a green cream to tone down and even out the rosiness. Classic orange and blue is a favourite combination of mine, and chocolate and rust are two smudgy colours that are comfortable in each other's company. Rust goes well with warmer blue tones, whereas salmon's opposite is an eau-de-nil. Cardinal purple makes for a striking contrast.

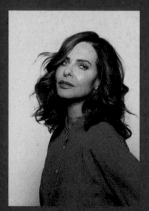
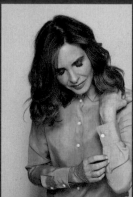
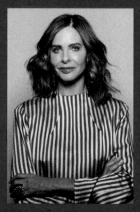

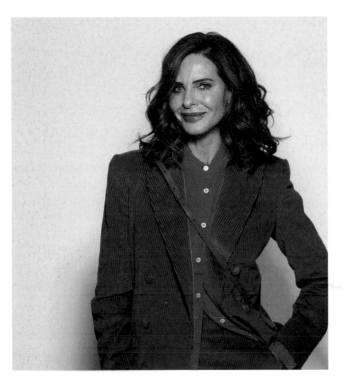

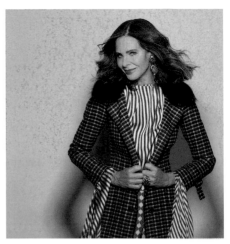

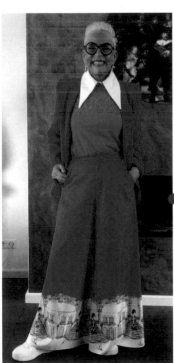

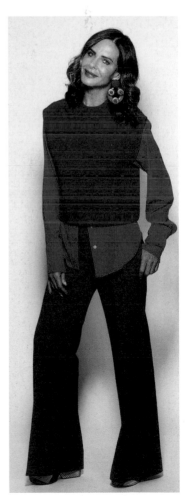

SYLVIA

A glorious statement orange outfit which is lifted by the statement collar, casual trainers and a pop of pink.

RED FAMILY

Red is bold, intentional and eye-catching. It's an expression of confidence - and most women know instinctively if they suit it or not. A red dress is a statement and something that has been elevated to iconic status in classic Hollywood movies. It's the easiest colour to wear if you are a classic cool blonde or deep toned and dark eyed - think Grace Kelly or Lupita Nyong'o. But what about the rest of us ...?

- If you are cool, you will likely suit a blue red or a raspberry red. Cool/neutrals will add a clear true red to this.

- Neutrals may be able to dabble with the shade that works for the cool or warm/neutrals, but may find clear red is best.

- Those with warm/neutral tones should try tomato shades, and if you are warm, a deep, muted autumn red can work.

The issue with red is that whatever your colour code, your skin tone and hair colour will play a big part in what works for you. If you have a pinky red undertone to your skin, and particularly if you have acne or rosacea, you may well find you just don't want to wear it. Some of us will find that power and confidence comes from another colour.

Whatever red you wear, please don't wear it with black. It will spoil the whole party. I could honestly write an essay about this but instead I will urge you to try it with metallics, with white, with navy, pink or orange - or by itself in all its glory.

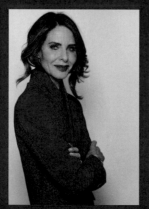
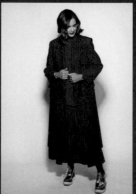
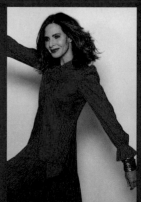

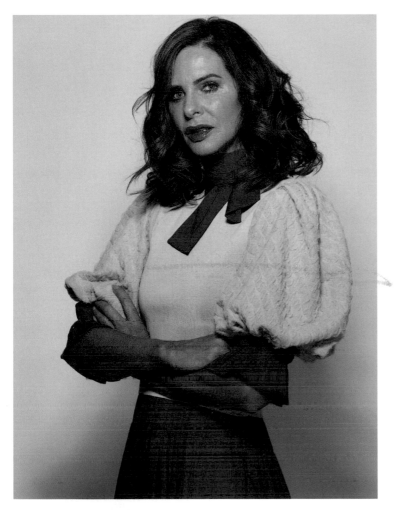

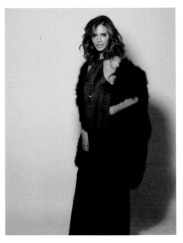

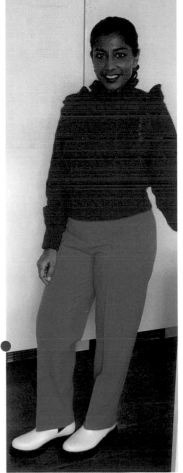

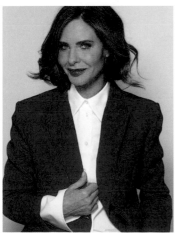

ANJANA

This is one of my favourite colour combinations, the colours are so vibrant when placed together.

Everyone can wear purple. I am being very loose with the term 'purple family', as I don't have enough pages! But for now, this includes burgundy, aubergine and plum, as well as classic lilac, purple and fuchsia. Purple is a wonderfully strong, powerful colour and there is a reason it was the colour used by the suffragettes and now on International Women's Day.

- If you are cool or cool/neutral, lilac and cold burgundy will suit you.

- If you are a neutral, you will look best in a true purple.

- For those who are warm or warm/neutral, a purple that is plum in tone will be your shade.

Burgundy, aubergine and plum can all be worn as alternatives to black as they are more versatile than you might think. But these are colours that are really killed by black.

You can tell which colours are friends because they bring a richness to each other. If you have something burgundy in your wardrobe, take it out and place it against something black. Now try it against something orange, fuchsia, navy or power blue. It's a completely different colour when it's allowed to play with its friends.

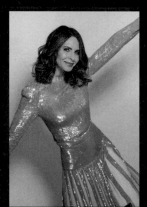
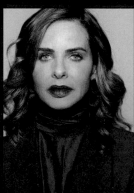
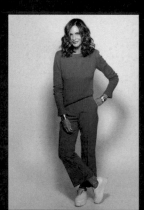

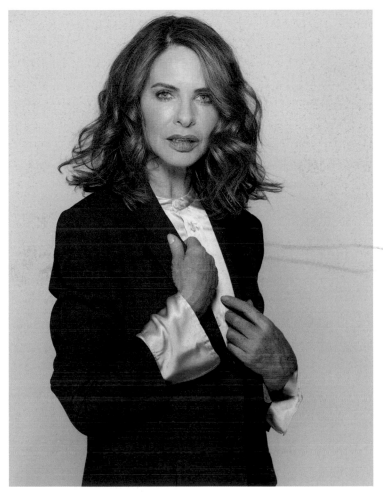

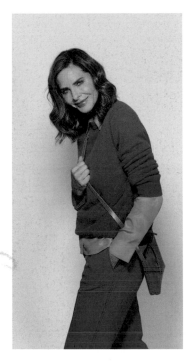

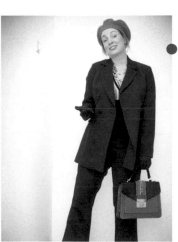

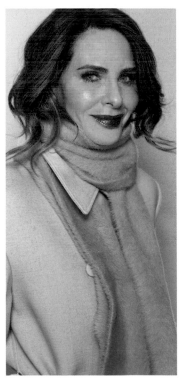

BETTINA

I love the way that Bettina has taken opposite ends of the colour spectrum and paired them together with the right tone. The yellow accessories are wonderful with the rich purple; she is having fun with this outfit.

BLUE FAMILY

We think of blue as a calming colour, but strong blues - like an air force or royal blue - can also feel quite powerful, while the brightest, sunniest blues make us think of holidays and freedom. It's one of the broadest colours in terms of the number of shades and it's a colour almost everyone can wear.

- If you are in the cool family, blue is very much your friend. Midnight, cobalt, royal blue, cerulean and indigo will likely feature heavily in your wardrobe.

- If you are a neutral, you will look best in clean blues, rather than anything bright or dirty. So aqua, azure, cornflower, slate or denim.

- For those who are warm, blue probably won't be your strongest colour but those shades at the teal end of the spectrum will work for you. Try a turquoise or an aquamarine. Blues with a greyish tone can also work.

Getting blues to go together are tricky. To wear blue tones together, they need to come from the same temperature family, for example cool blues don't look good with warm blues. Whereas French navy and pastel blue looks classic and fresh. Blue plays fabulously with other shades. I love a darker blue or cobalt with orange. Burgundy with pastel blue is a good combination if you are a cool, while plum and aquamarine is stunning if you are warm in tone.

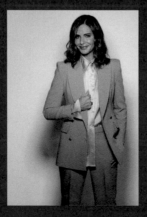 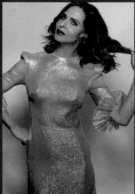 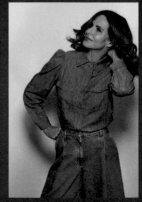

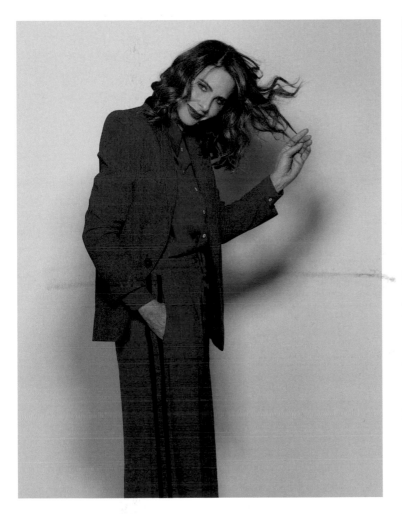

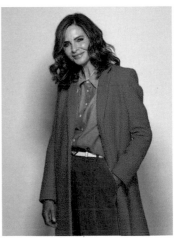

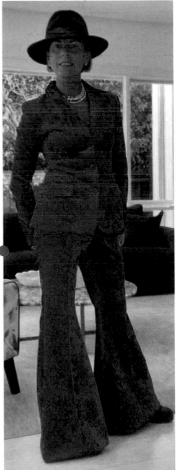

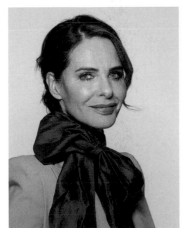

ROSEMARY

The velvet suit is a great statement outfit and offers up the opportunity for some daytime luxury.

GREEN FAMILY

I realised when I was doing the photoshoot for this book that I don't wear much green. Green is a very broad family from mint to pea, as well as emerald to forest, and khaki to bottle. There are many great contrasting shades you can wear. But interestingly, as greens are very specific individual shades, it can be difficult to mix shades together.

- If you are cool, you will look wonderful in mint green, bright emerald and coolest dark green.

- If you are cool/neutral, wear apple, pea green and khaki with cool undertones.

- If you are a neutral, you will look best in forest, fern and leafy greens.

- For those who are warm/neutral, you will suit warm khakis which are green and brown with a yellow tone.

- If you are warm, you will look fabulous in teal.

If you do want to try mixing shades of green together, a good start is to use those that are used in camouflage colourways as inspiration. If you love the colour green, khaki and olive can work as good alternatives to black, as they are fairly neutral.

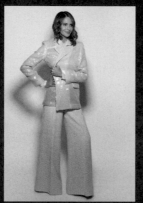
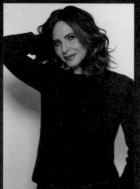
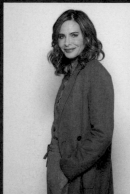

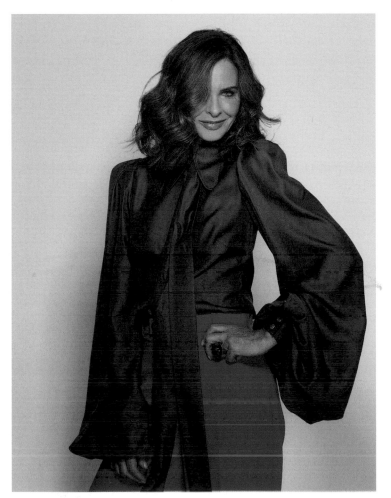

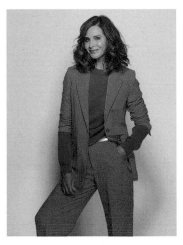

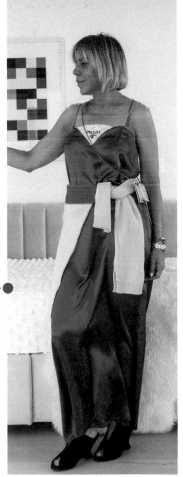

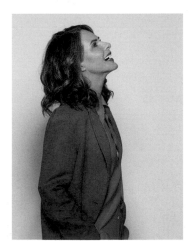

RACHEL

A wonderful combination of the luxurious green silk and soft pink.

YELLOW FAMILY

Yellow is a fabulous colour that projects energy to those around you. I bet you notice people respond to you slightly differently when you are wearing yellow.

- At the cool end of the yellow scale is the neons, turning into the pale lemons.

- If you are a neutral, you can pick from the middle of the yellow, so from the stronger lemons up into daffodil. A peaches-and-cream complexion suits a lemon yellow or a pale pastel.

- The warms among us, particularly if you have caramel skin and a warmth in your hair, will go for daffodil to saffron.

Yellow is such a fascinating colour. Just a tweak of your hair colour can make a difference to your very best yellow and send you sliding up or down the yellow scale. The spectrum of yellows is much shorter than you find in the blues or greens, but yellow knows what it wants. Down in the cool shades, silver or white are a wonderful addition. But up in to daffodil and beyond, you could wear a soft gold. Conversely, a warm-based leopard print is wonderful with saffron but will not play at all with neon. If you absolutely must, you can wear neon with black. But if you're looking for a neutral for all the other shades, try a grey.

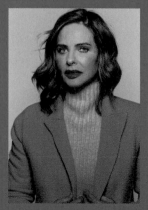
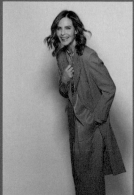
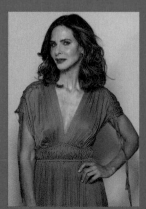

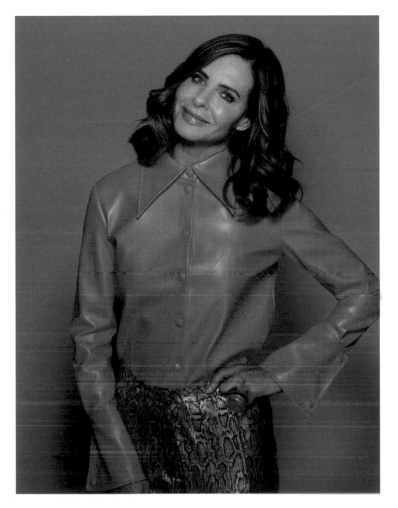

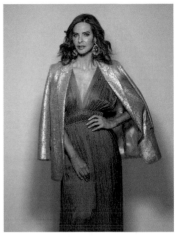

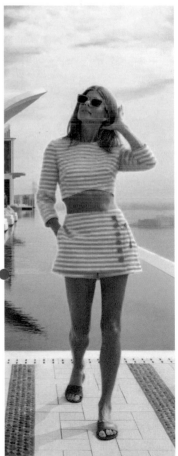

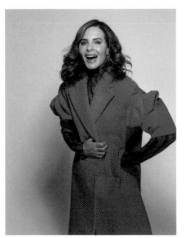

LEAH

Yellow always brings such confidence and presence to an outift. The two piece element of this outfit works beautifully.

NEON

Neons are impactful and electric. They are completely synthetic colours that don't exist in nature. In a pantone book, neons get their own page together, away from the other colour families. Neons are exciting partly because they make their own rules. When I am styling a woman, I sometimes don't know how she will look in neon, what will work best for her, until I try it out.

- If you are a cool or a cool/neutral you will find it easiest to wear neon. The people who it works best for are those with black skin and grey undertones or those who have a very big contrast between their skin, hair and eye colour. If this is you, you probably already know you look great in neon.

- If you are neutral, you can wear neon. You just have to check against your hair colour, i.e. if you are a slightly warmer blonde you might prefer a pink neon over an orange one.

- If you are warmer toned, the acidity that defines neon might be too much for you if you wear a lot of it.

- Everyone can wear some neon to bring an outfit to life.

I will happily wear top-to-toe neon and I have been told I look like a highlighter pen many times! To walk around in colours that were purposely created to draw the eye is the ultimate expression of confidence. But everyone can grab some of this energy for themselves, even if it's just a flash of neon on a belt or shoe. I love neon and tweed because the clash of this traditional fabric with the modernity of neon creates something that feels very exciting.

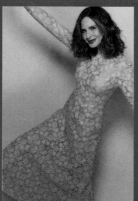
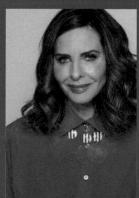
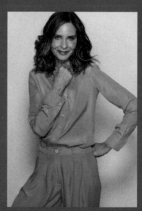

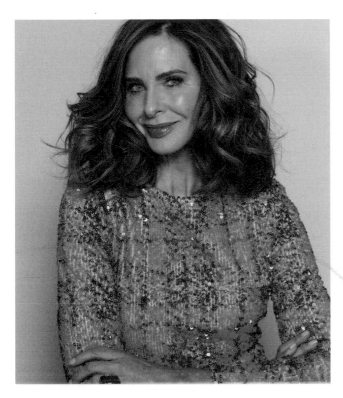

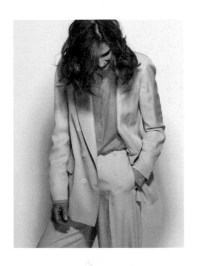

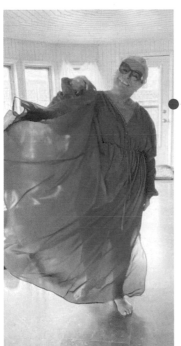

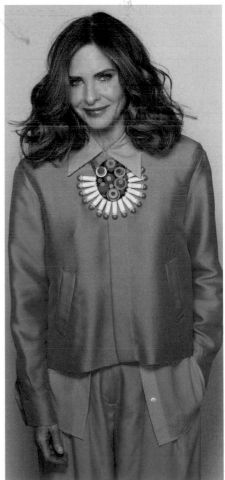

MANNY

Manny always inspires me with her choice of colour, and this outfit embodies everything that is fabulous about neon. I also love the finishing touch of the perspex neon pink glasses!

METALLICS

We've talked already about the surprising versatility of a sequinned jacket but even if you don't want to go that far, metallics are an important part of any wardrobe for their ability to light you up and bring you alive. On a day that you feel tired, they will lift your complexion.

- If you are cool or cool/neutral, silver is best.

- If you are a neutral, you can wear any shade.

- If you're a warm/neutral or warm, choose gold.

Never underestimate the transformative power of metallics. A grey suit that looks rather businessy is a whole different thing with a frivolous silver top underneath. A black dress with a statement gold belt or a necklace that sits on the high neckline is glamorous and confident rather than workday. And you absolutely can wear metallics during the day. I particularly like an everyday shape in a metallic – for example, imagine a simple round neck jumper in grey with a navy blazer and jeans. Now think about that jumper in silver. It just adds something extra, elevating what would otherwise be a straightforward classic look.

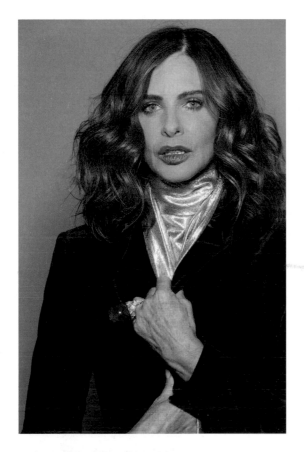

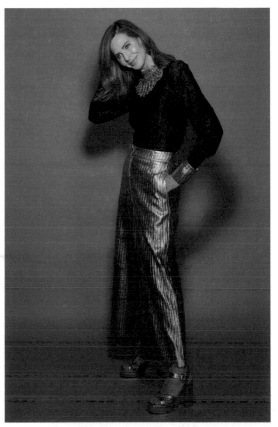

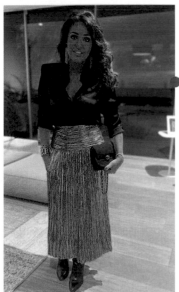

LEILA

What a gorgeous skirt, with an incredibly flattering shape. I love that Leila has picked out accents of the gold in her jewellery and the buckle of her bag too.

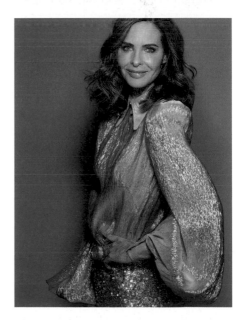

NAVY

Navy is my black. I have a lot of it in my wardrobe. It is softer but still stylish, classic and modern all at the same time. But it can be more challenging as, unlike black, there are many shades and some will be better for you than others.

- If your colour code is a cool or cool/neutral, then you will find it easy to wear a classic navy with a grey undertone.

- If you are a neutral, you will likely be able to wear navies from across the middle of the spectrum.

- If you're a warm/neutral or warm, you won't want your navy too cool.

Different navies work with different colours but all are versatile and get along with other neutrals. I particularly love navy and white in a stripe as it's such a clean, casual look. The only thing that is tricky is that not all of what we refer to generally as navy will cooperate. To wear navy on navy, you are looking for the same underlying tone. It doesn't matter so much if two navies are lighter or darker, as long as they have the same amount of grey or purple. Navies that are warmer or dirtier will fight.

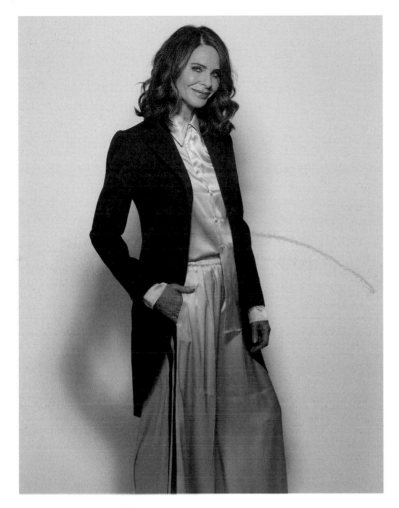

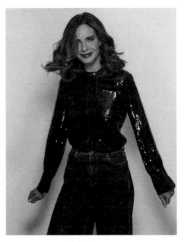

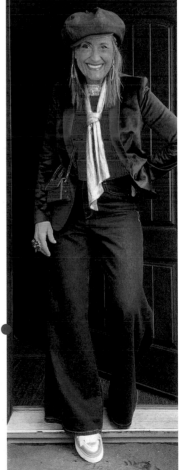

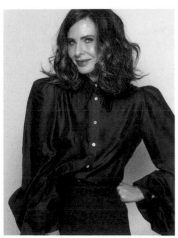

TAMMY

Tammy has combined one of my favourite shades with navy here, which is orange. And as she is cool toned, she has brought everything together with a silver scarf.

BLACK

Let's get this out of the way: I do of course wear black – it's chic, it's elegant, it's classic. Black can empower you and give you strength against the unknowns of a day. However, I have realised that I should only wear black when I feel at my absolute best, not when I feel tired because it will sap what energy I do have.

I think 25 per cent of people can wear black with no makeup and look amazing (these are cool toned people). Another 50 per cent need makeup to wear black, and 25 per cent probably shouldn't wear black at all – or certainly not near their face.

Dull, flat black is draining, while fresh, sharply cut black can be chic and glamorous. So how can we bring black to life?

Texture is key. Something that catches the light and pushes it back out – a sequin, fake fur, velvet – has a different effect to a dull black that sucks up the light. Black with metallic running through it gives an instant lift.

White accents are useful to wake up the black. Introduce white via collars, sleeves or accessories like a white trainer.

Most of us have a black dress in the wardrobe, so what can you do to lift this? Consider putting a shirt underneath, as the collar means the black isn't against your skin. Think about how black and white work together in the form of checks, stripes, polka dot and houndstooth.

You can wear black with navy, white tones, grey, brown (leopard print), gold and silver. But it is very draining for some colours – it not only washes out some people's skin tone, it wrings out colours like blush, pale yellows, lavenders …

If you wear a lot of black, do you need a red lip to bring attention back to your face and stop yourself from disappearing into it, or are you better off perfecting a fabulous smokey eye and a neutral lip (which is my preferred way when I wear black)?

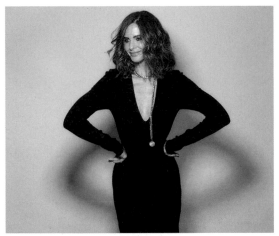

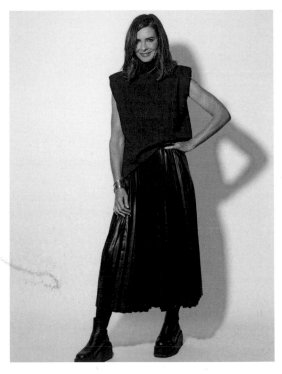

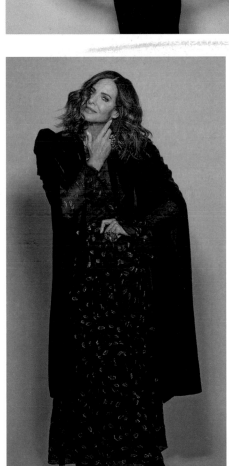

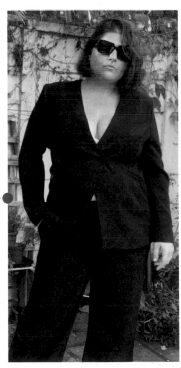

CHLOE

Chloe looks incredible in this outfit as the tailoring offers a great shape and she is wearing a black that is not too harsh.

How to wear print...

There is something so eye-catching and irresistible about a beautifully designed print. When deciding if a print is right for you, these are the things to consider.

Is the print wearing you?

If you look in the mirror and, from two metres away, see the print before you see your face, then it is wearing you. That may be because the pattern is too big or there are too many colours too near your face. Some prints we can only carry off if we are wearing a lot of makeup, particularly a strong lip colour.

How big and dense is the size of the print?

Fuller figured women can often carry off a big, bold print that would swamp someone more petite. There is more space for the pattern to repeat so you get a sense of it, which allows you to really own it. It's also harder to wear a bold print if you have very delicate features, though polka dot may look good on you.

Which part of your body will it emphasise?

If you are a larger busted woman who prefers to play down her top half then you may not feel comfortable wearing a print over your breasts, whereas a print in a trouser or skirt topped with a plain blouse will rebalance you.

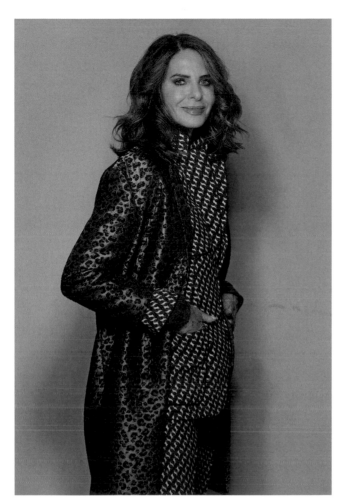

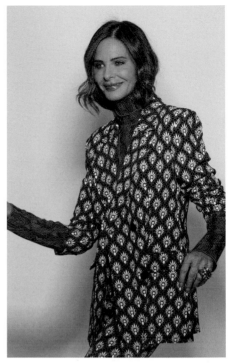

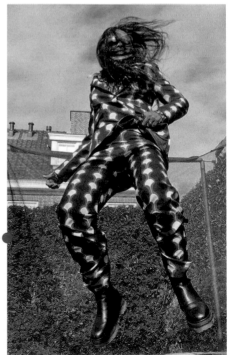

MARITIA

The most glorious colourful, vibrant and joyful suit that Maritia has made her own. The chunky boot looks great with this outfit.

Can you echo the shape of the print in an earring or accessory?

Try to bring out different elements of the print in different places to create a sense of flow. Avoid being too matchy-matchy, as you want it to seem effortless. I have a palm leaf skirt that I love to wear with yellow palm earrings as it brings the whole thing together.

Can you create a family of prints?

To mix two or more prints, they need to have a relationship and proportionality. It's much harder to mix a big print with something delicate. It helps if they share at least two colours. If prints only share one colour, they need a belt to bring them together. If you start to layer the prints, such as adding a bag or scarf in yet another pattern but in the same colour family, the excess and confidence makes it work.

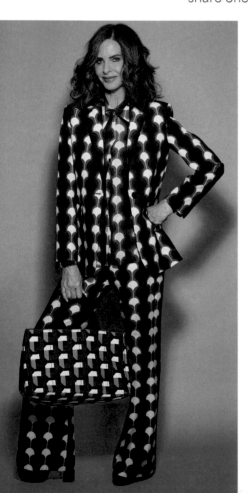

Can you mix black and white prints?

Yes! Just pay attention to what sort of white is in each, as cream against white will look dirty.

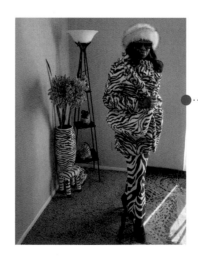

ANDRALEE

Print galore! This is a great example of mixing black and white prints – and in your home accessories too!

ASK YOURSELF

1 Is there a simple way for you to introduce some pattern or print into your outfit?

2 Are you afraid of pattern clash?

3 Do you think you can't wear print at all?

4 Do you have any favourite accessories you can use as a starting point for exploring patterns?

CHALLENGE YOURSELF

1 One of the subtlest ways to try out pattern clash is with a shoe. If you are wearing a patterned dress, it can feel natural to go for a neutral shoe. But a slight clash in the same colours can make for a fun twist.

2 Taking the print away from our face and choosing a colour from it that works next to our skin is the most flattering way to wear print.

3 If you don't normally wear print, don't rule out animal print. They work for anyone if you get the right tone and size of pattern.

4 Don't be scared of pattern clash. I know a lot depends on personality, but if you feel like you are carrying something off then you probably are. You may surprise yourself with what you dare to wear.

The essentials

If you have a version of the items listed below, then it will give you a solid foundation on which you can then build your personal style.

1 White trainer
Nothing makes outfits feel fresher than a stacked white trainer.

2 Metallic shoe
So hard working that you won't need many other shoes.

3 White jacket
You will wear this so much more than you might think.

4 Breton T-shirt
An easy-to-wear classic that can be styled up and in a neckline that suits.

5 The perfect white T-shirt
With your best arm shape/length and neckline, and fitted.

6 A great coat
Don't be conservative and feel this has to go with everything.

7 A flattering dress
In the right colour and shape for you, this can take you from day to night.

8 The perfect shape jeans
The holy grail, if sometimes a pain to shop for.

The non-essential essentials

Let me introduce you to non-essential essentials. They are the things that bring you joy. You might even consider them to be frivolous and may not have thought to wear them before. But when you find ones that work for you, they will elevate what you wear and turn a jean and a top, for example, into an outfit.

Non-essential essentials bring the clothes you wear them with to life. They may be noisier than what you usually wear and so you might feel hesitant to try them, thinking 'Is this really me?' But they are at the heart of fearless dressing because they make you stand out rather than blend in.

I love it when women tell me they had never worn a sequin before but then stepped outside their comfort zone, bought a sequin jacket and now wear it all the time. Because when you embrace this concept, you'll realise how hard working non-essential essentials can be. We dress to look good and to feel confident, but we can have fun too. So in this section you'll find eight of my favourite non-essential essentials and what they do. I want to give you permission, or an excuse, if you need it, to take a risk and push the boat out.

Have a look in your wardrobe. What are your non-essential essentials? How can you challenge yourself to embrace them and let them take you further on your style journey?

These items are at the heart of fearless dressing

SEQUIN

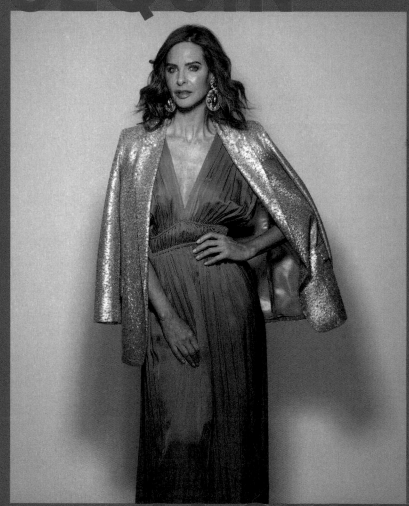

JACKET

This is a marvellous example of a non-essential essential because a sequin jacket can change the way we feel and has so many more uses than you might assume. It is a brilliant piece to elevate any outfit and should be bought as a lifetime investment.

It brings glamour

Sequins add glamour to a casual look and will make a T-shirt and jeans go anywhere - the answer to a 'I don't know what to wear' smart-casual invite. While at the same time being perfect over an evening dress that won't love your work-day coat.

Sequins reflect light

You might be worried that sequins will bulk you out. In fact, because of the way they move they do the opposite. People don't notice your figure in sequins – they notice you sparkling as you enter the room and want to talk to you. The way sequins reflect the light back up is also a wonderful antidote to a hungover, jetlagged or tired face.

Buy the right shade

Buy the metallic that's right for your tones (see page 15). If you start with your perfect neutral, you can build up to other colours.

Dress up or down

Bear in mind that while sequins are fabulous against fabric, such as over a top, wearing them against your skin with nothing underneath is what takes it into nighttime. And if you are trying to make the look more appropriate for the day, try a more neutral makeup.

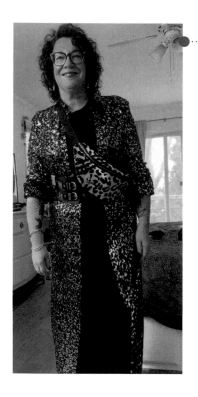

KERRY

*I love this version
of a sequin jacket.
It immediately brings
confidence and light to
a black outfit. The belt
cinched in at the waist
is an excellent addition.*

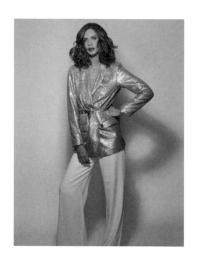

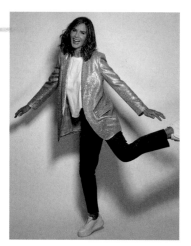

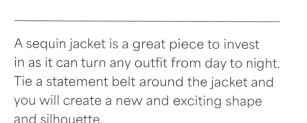

A sequin jacket is a great piece to invest
in as it can turn any outfit from day to night.
Tie a statement belt around the jacket and
you will create a new and exciting shape
and silhouette.

The right shade of sequin for your tone
(see page 15) can add an eye-catching
element to any dark or single colour outfit.

I love to wear a sequin jacket with
a soft trouser with a great drape. The
juxtaposition of fabrics adds a real feel
of luxury to an outfit.

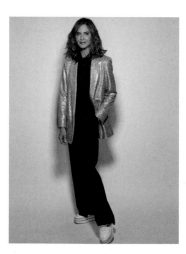

METALLIC

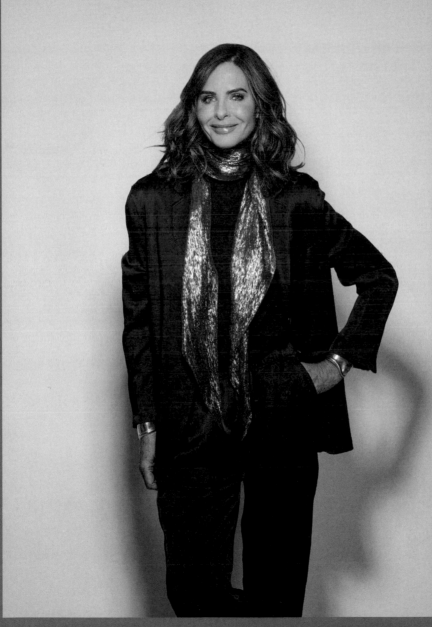

SCARF

This could be a metallic or a sequin scarf. You will find
this has so many uses it could be on the list of essentials.
I appreciate a metallic scarf isn't always easy to find,
so you can use a sequin scarf for this type of look instead.

From day to night

With a red lip, it is the perfect piece to add to an outfit if you
are going straight from work to the restaurant or bar. And it
will fit into your handbag so you can quickly put it on en-route.

Choose the right tone

It is important to pick the tone to best suit your skin. It will be
gold if you are a warm and silver if you are a cool.

Wear it in a multitude of ways

It's the flourish that upgrades a simple dress and jacket and will
go with almost any print that works for you. You don't just have
to wear it as a scarf, either, as it can double up as a belt.

It will reflect the light

All metallics will work hard in your wardrobe but wearing them
right next to your face has a similar effect to sequins - it throws
the light back, wakes you up and illuminates you.

NICOLETTE

*This is a really cool and laid back look.
It has fabulous rock chic elements to it.*

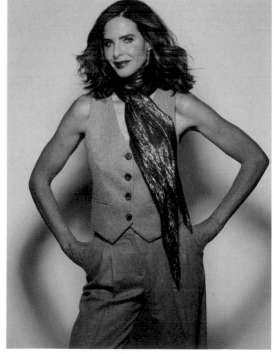

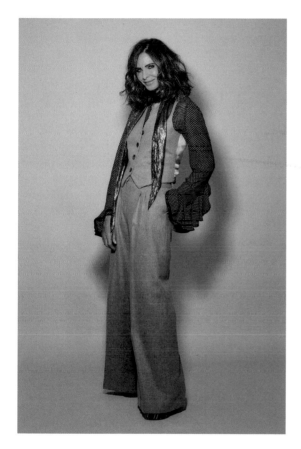

A metallic scarf is a very simple piece to introduce to an outfit and it can be tucked in your bag for any occassion. You could twist the scarf around once and do it up in the middle, in a pussybow; or you could wear it draped in a 1970's fashion; or you could tie it round your waist as a belt.

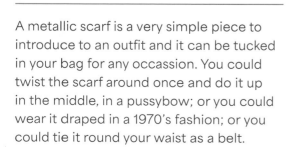

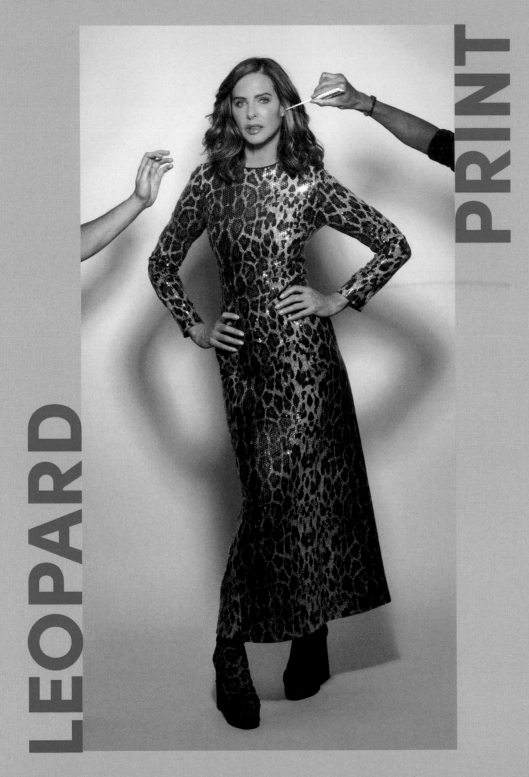

LEOPARD

PRINT

Leopard print has gone from an occasional trend that would flit on and off the catwalk to a classic that you see in the shops every season.

It's a neutral

Even if you can't wear print you can probably wear leopard. People are often surprised when I tell them it is a neutral, but it is, and it can be worn with pretty much anything. It is also bold and playful, making it a key non-essential essential. Leopard print can be layered with leopard. The trick is to keep the size of the print similar and to have a mixture of one of the base tones equally represented in all prints. Otherwise, just go for it.

Start small

I love my leopard coat as the structure works well with the print. And it goes with almost everything. But if you are not sure where to start begin with something smaller. A bag, a shoe or a scarf will always look chic and will make friends with many items in your wardrobe. If you've not worn the print before you might be surprised by how often you find yourself reaching for it.

Select the right tone

If you are a cool or a cool/neutral, you are looking for a cooler-toned, almost grey-based leopard. If you are a warm/neutral or warm then the classic warm beige and tan tones will work.

Dress up or down

Matching makeup to leopard will depend on where you are wearing it. If the print is next to your face, a neutral lip looks chic with a smokey eye, but equally a red lip can really make it pop.

Leopard is where I layer most. It is also brilliant at pulling an outfit together and disguising when two other items might not quite match, i.e. two different types of sequins.

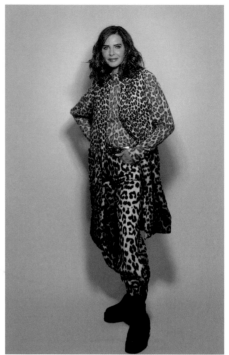

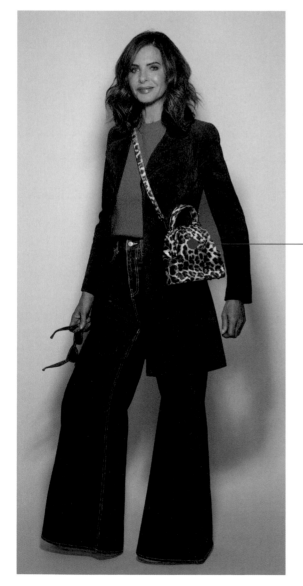

Consider starting with an accessory like a leopard print bag. This will just switch up a classic jean and suede jacket outfit.

This shows different textures of print, but there is a continuity in the base colours.

DANIELA

I love the combination of leopard prints, with the addition of the bright pop of colour from the orange jacket.

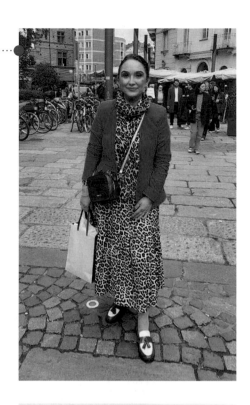

PINKY

This outfit is full of confidence! Pinky shows no fear and completely embraces the beauty of leopard print.

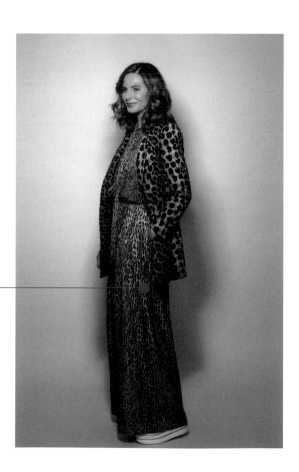

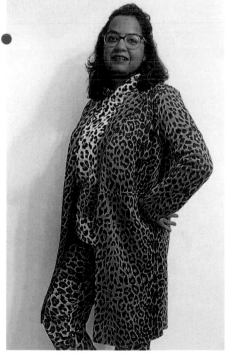

METALLIC

BAG

If you are not someone who owns a lot of bags, a metallic version is exactly what you need as you will get so much use out of it. Choose a metallic bag that will work with your tones (see page 15). You will then be able to pair it with anything in your wardrobe. Rarely do we leave the house without a bag on our arm, and a metallic bag can be one of the most practical items that you will come to own.

It is modern

A metallic bag will give an instant lift to a classic outfit and make it feel fresh and modern.

Wear it with print

If you are someone who likes to wear a lot of print then a metallic will go with almost everything, meaning you can sidestep defaulting to the standard black bag that can suck the life out of colours.

Adds daytime glamour

A metallic bag might seem too glitzy for the daytime but it is all in the shape and structure - it needs to have more structure to make it feel more suitable for the daytime.

It works with every outfit

If you are going out in either the evening or day, or you are going on a trip and only have room to pack one bag, you never have to think 'which bag shall I take?' as it will go with everything.

What I love about this bag is that it can be a cross-body bag, or I tuck the straps in and it can be a clutch. It is in my perfect shade of a matt silver, so it goes with every single daytime outfit that I own. I can then just put the strap in and take the outfit from day to night.

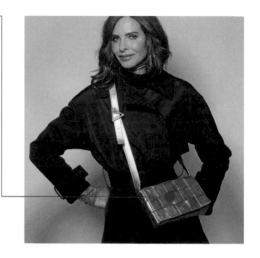

This tote bag is the perfect size for all that I need in the office. I can put it with any outfit and it doesn't matter if it goes through a bit of wear and tear during the day.

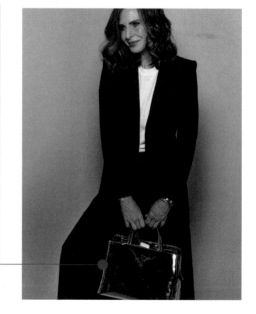

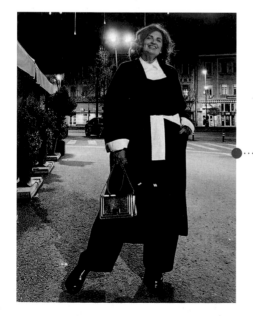

EVA

This is a an excellent choice, Eva has avoided choosing a bag that is black, which would have flattened the outfit. The clean lines of the layering and matt silver works perfectly with this outfit.

STATEMENT

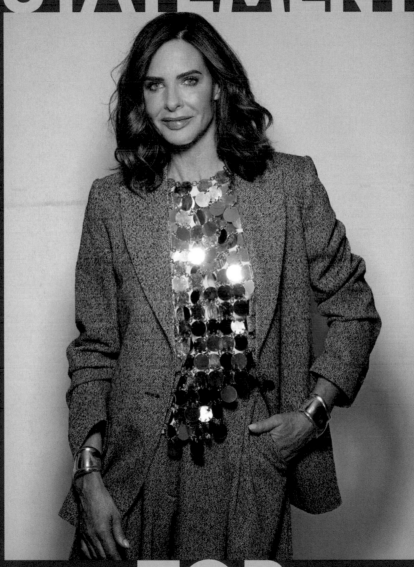

TOP

A statement top is that item that can bring drama to a classic outfit. That may well be through the fabric itself, the colour, the sleeve, an amazing cuff, some contrast piping or through a particularly architectural shape. The point is that it does all the talking and you need nothing (or little) else.

There are variations

A statement top can be sequins, or bright in colour or pattern. It is any top that brings life to an outfit, and can mean different things to different people.

It is easy to wear

A statement top might be something that pushes you to the edge of your comfort zone because you feel like you are only just getting away with it. But it will project an air of confidence while being surprisingly easy to wear because you don't need many accessories or layers.

It is for any shape

If you are a big-boobed woman you might have become used to not drawing attention to your top half and think the statement top is not for you. When in fact a big sleeve can balance out a large bust and look fabulous.

Don't stick to black

Importantly, if the statement is in the print then choose a colour from the print to wear on your bottom half. Don't just default to black as this will cut you in half and suck the life from the other colours. Try it now – get your print top and put it against different colours in your wardrobe.

Day

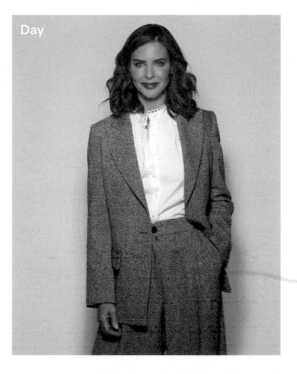

Night

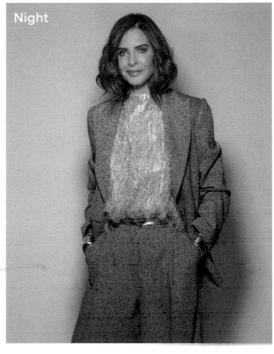

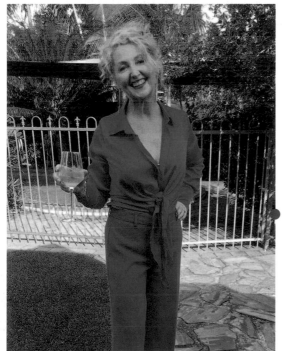

People either love or hate this shirt! The joy of this statement top it that it can go with anything, including a grey suit as it works tonally. There is nothing better than upping the ante with a bit of sequin or sparkle and reinvigorating a basic suit.

AMANDA

This statement top adds drama through the fabric, shape and colour. Amanda has created a cohesive outfit by pairing with a trouser in a complementary tone.

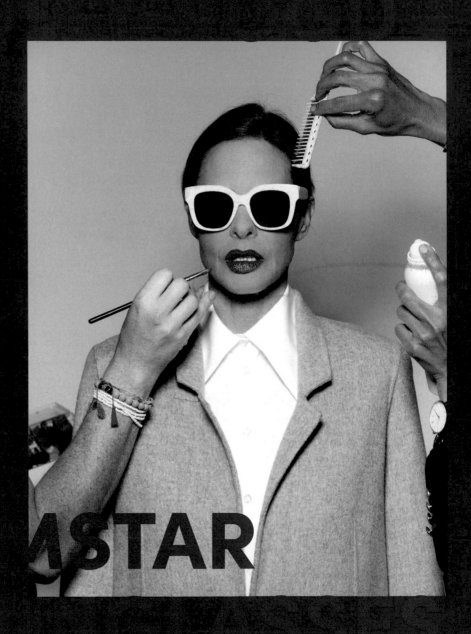

ASTAR

These are not the usual Ray Bans or simple chic cat's eye for every day. These are the sunglasses that you put on, walk down the street and they give you a certain swagger. Sunglasses are all about the shape and the colour.

They bring joy

There is nothing sensible about these glasses. You don't need them but they will bring you joy (so actually maybe they are needed ...). They may be quirky and unusual, which will challenge you to live up to their appeal.

An easy twist

Hollywood film star sunglasses are a great entry-level non-essential essential as they are easy to wear and need no commitment - they are just one small detail that you take off when you go inside and don't have to wear all day. They really are the perfect fun accessory.

There is a version for everyone

There will be a version of the Hollywood film star sunglasses for everyone, you just need to find yours. Go to page 207 if you want some general tips on choosing glasses - however, I would say that with Hollywood film star sunglasses, if they make you feel fabulous then the rule of whether they suit your face shape just goes out the window.

Play with colour

Not only can you select statement shapes, but you can add drama and interest with colourful frames too.

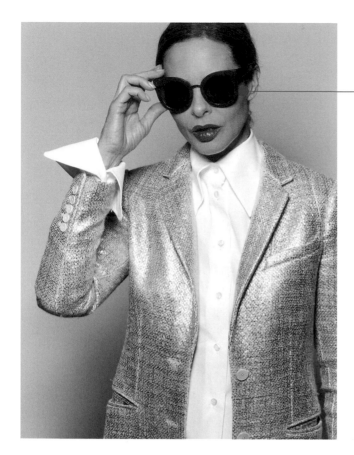

I love navy blue, and this is just a slightly lighter shade which suits my face better, as it is slightly softer. The shape lifts my face as the glasses don't come down at all.

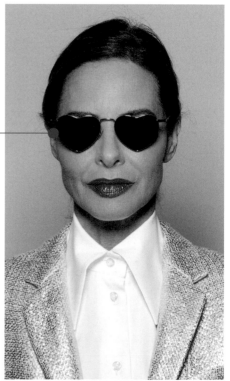

I look at this photo now and I am not quite sure of them, because I can see my eyebrow above one of them, which show they are probably a little bit too small for my face. However, I adore heart-shaped sunglasses, and we should all be able to bring moments of joy into our wardrobe.

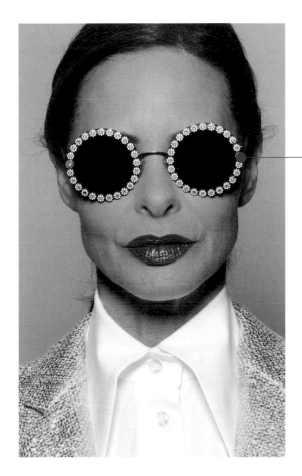

My Dolce & Gabbana sunglasses.
I cannot believe I still have these after
10 years, they are my most treasured
sunglasses. I wear them most of the
days that the sun is shining, so cost
per wear is getting better …

SAMANTHA

*Choosing a shape which
lifts her heart shaped face,
and a very cool hat, gives
her a look that says 'I am a
confident woman, enjoying
myself on holiday.'*

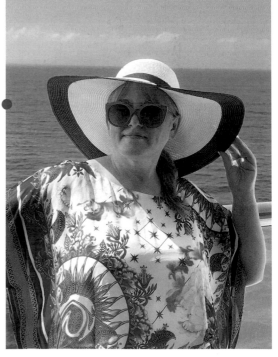

NEON

ACCESSORY

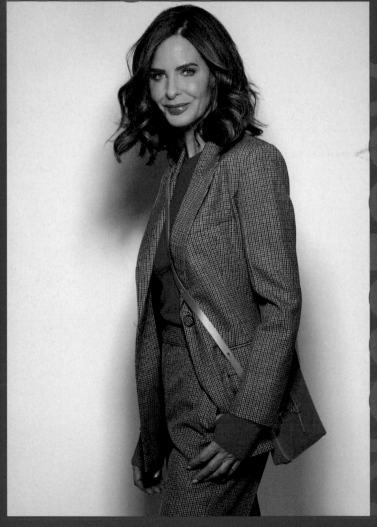

You might never have considered neon because you think it is just for children's television presenters or 1980 ravers. I am here to tell you that neon is one of the ultimate non-essential essentials that – in some form – can, and should, be worn by everyone. This will lift any look and is something we can all try more often.

It brings life

Even a hint of neon will instantly take the dust off an outfit, change it up and make it more modern. If an item feels a bit boring or old fashioned and you need to wake it up, neon will do this. Take neon and tweed, for example. If you're wearing a hit of bright neon it can't fail to energise you. It is not possible to slump around in neon.

Choose the right tone

Deciding which neon you are is the first step. The coolest tone of yellow is neon. It has no warmth but it is bright. If your colour code is warm, you might be better in pink neon. Bright orange is often best with neutral skin tones.

Start away from your face

If neon is far away from the colours you suit, don't start in earrings or jewellery, start further away from your face with the flash of a trainer or the accent of a bag.

Small accents

Consider hints of neon that poke out of your clothing. You could wear a block colour jumper, but underneath you have the sleeve and the tails of a neon shirt poking out. This will give a modern element to an outfit which might otherwise feel classic.

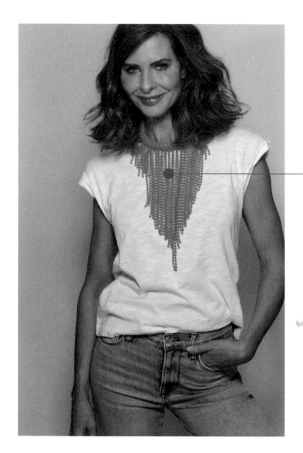

I have had this H&M necklace for about 15 years and cost per wear is now minimal. It changes so many outfits. I can wear it over a smart dress to make it look more casual and over a T-shirt to elevate.

The big neon bag is a statement piece. I don't know how I have managed to hold onto it – Lyla is always trying to steal it from me!

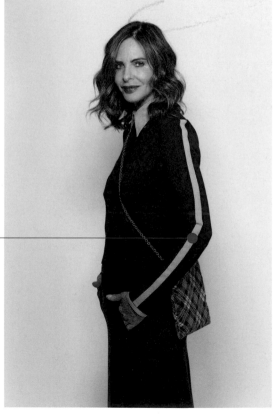

Here I have given multiple examples of how a flash of neon can peek out of any outfit and make it look original. Neon is brilliant for making dark outfits or suits look cool, a little bit of neon can change everything. It will make it look fresh and give you a completely new outlook on life.

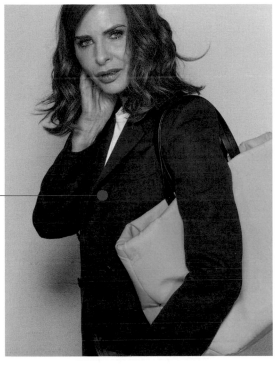

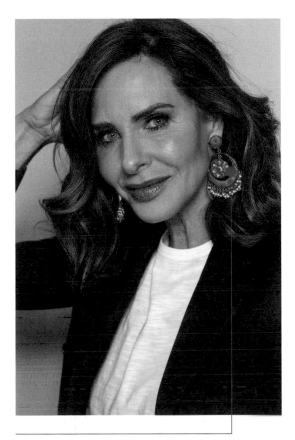

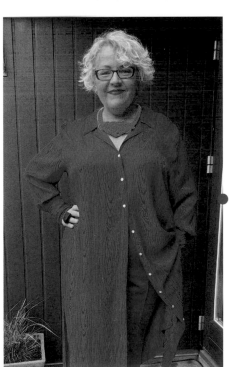

The strong neon pink of this earring is balanced by the softer orange. I am therefore able to wear a strong makeup look with it and it won't fight.

TINE

Bold, bright and wonderful! What a joyful elevation to the stunning blue outfit.

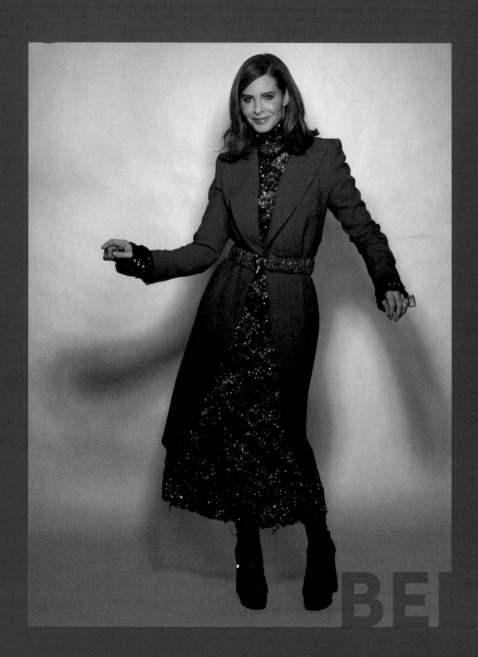

BELT

This is one of the simplest and quickest ways to elevate an outfit. There's got to be a belt in every woman's life that she can put on over the most boring black dress and immediately it looks like the jewel of the outfit. They can be affordable and take up minimal space in the cupboard, which means you are able to get a few different ones to create variation.

It creates shape

A belt can be an incredibly beautiful feature that draws the eye to what is generally the narrowest part of a woman's body.

Choose the right width

The width of the belt will depend on the length of your torso and the length of the dress you are wearing. If you are short bodied a narrower belt will be better, though if you are wearing a long dress you can usually get away with something wider because there is enough fabric below it that the belt isn't cutting you off right in the middle.

Buckle shape is key

Women with a larger bust will suit a round buckle but if you are very angular a rectangular fastening may well be better.

Day to night

A statement belt is one of the simplest and fastest ways to transform an outfit from day to night. A statement belt has that extra punch. It might have an amazing buckle, it might be made from metal - in silver or gold - or have pearls, but it becomes a piece of jewellery that will add interest and focus to your outfit.

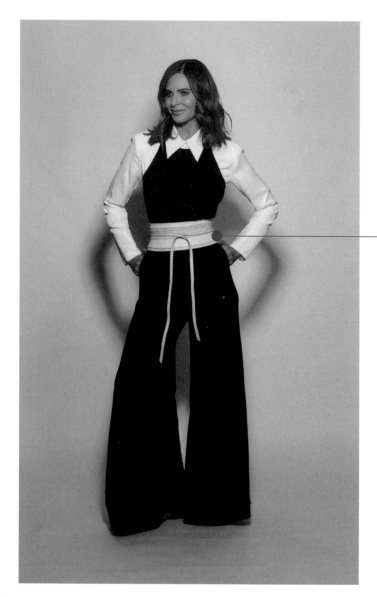

An Obi tie belt can be a very good waist cincher. You can get them in different depths. This white belt goes around your waist and pulls to the front. It is a way to really enhance your shape and they are typically slightly curved to give more emphasis to your waist.

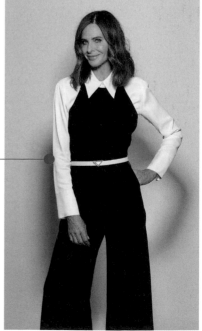

If you are short waisted, a thin belt is the perfect way to bring your waist in as a wide belt will go straight from your breast to your hip and hide your shape. It will also bring in a loose summer dress to give your body shape more emphasis.

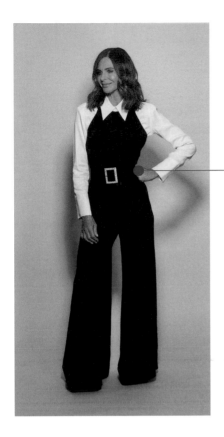

A belt with a statement buckle is great if you are short waisted or petite. It will pull you in but allows the flow of your torso not to be interrupted and therefore doesn't foreshorten your waist.

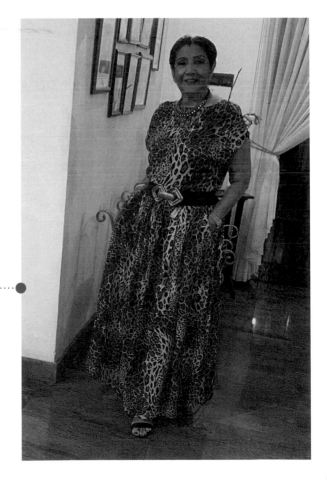

PAULINE

This is a fabulously eye-catching belt which creates a great shape in the dress.

How to layer...

I love to layer. Yes, it requires some thought but this is where we challenge ourselves to understand how items can work together in ways we may not have considered. Layering creates a confident look. It's also practical, as what you're wearing can take you through the day and be easily modified for the evening. There is a flow to it which is joyful to embrace and you will feel it when you are getting it right.

It does take more time to put a layered outfit together because you have to consider colour and length and flow all together, but it is practical and fun. Sure, we might usually avoid contrasting hem lengths in skirts and coats, but with soft layers the rules can absolutely change.

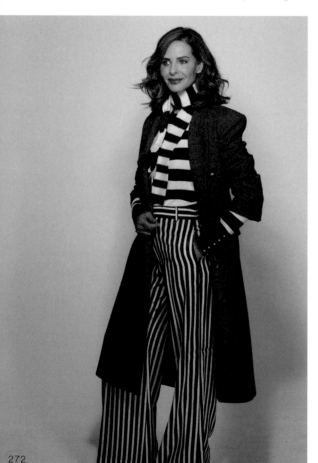

The concern lots of us have with layering is that it can add bulk. So to avoid that we are mainly looking for very thin layers – like a soft gilet or a long but light shirt.

A look works when each layer ends in the right place. Think about what you want to cover and where you want the eye to go. This creates an intentionality and flow, as opposed to a collection of long bits of fabric making you look elongated or smothered.

Don't forget to honour your shape. If you pay attention to your waist, and show an ankle or a wrist, then the contrast between these slim parts of you and the drape of soft layers will always be very flattering.

Remember the colours and tones involved are important – they need to co-operate with one another and not fight.

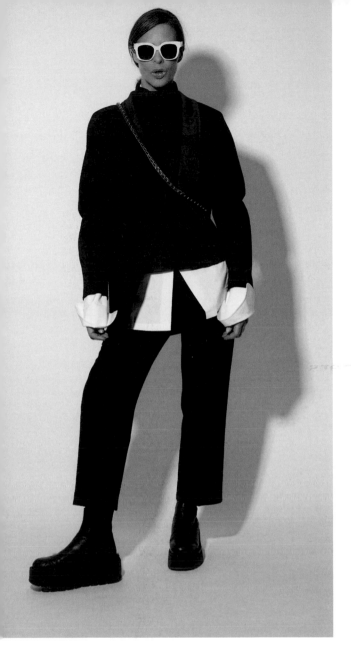

- A half-tuck of a top into a trouser is a great intro to layering. Soften where your top and bottom half meet, covering the join to bring them together.

- A thin gilet can go under a jacket, particularly helpful if the jacket is slightly short, hitting the wrong part of your bottom. Adding a thicker gilet over a coat – perhaps in fake fur – for warmth in winter means you don't need to wear a heavy coat you'll be carrying under your arm by lunchtime. A gilet over a jacket will make it a coat.

- Try a belt over layering to give the outfit structure.

- Wear trousers under skirts. Just think about where each layer finishes on your body and consider whether you need to be able to see your ankle below the trousers and dress. A light trouser under a kaftan is a very good, practical example of this. When you are walking around the city in the summer you might not want to wear a loose fitting beachy kaftan with slits up the side. But with trousers underneath and a wedge shoe, it is transformed into something else entirely.

Accessories to elevate every look

While clothes at their most basic get you covered up for the day, accessories are where we can express ourselves, experiment and fearlessly elevate what we have chosen to put on. Generally accessories don't go out of fashion, so they will be the pieces that will last longest in your wardrobe. They are a simple way to reinvigorate an outfit you are bored of wearing.

They are also about celebrating the bits of our bodies we love and feel confident about, as they draw the eye. Women with elegant ankles should have a fabulous collection of shoes. Those with an hourglass figure can celebrate that with a statement belt.

Accessories also tweak an outfit that isn't quite working the way you want. A statement necklace will offset a collar that doesn't sit quite right. A scarf will bring a pop of colour next to your face if you are feeling washed out.

They are so useful when you are travelling as they change up an outfit and don't take up space. A pair of earrings and a metallic scarf is perfect to liven up a neutral look and can take you from day to evening.

If you are not yet feeling fearless in your dressing, this is where you can easily challenge yourself first. Add just one element to your dressing and show your individuality through your accessory choice.

The right accessories make a wardrobe more wearable

Scarves

A scarf can bring colour up to your face, so they should always be in your best colours. If you are colour blocking, the right scarf will bring everything together. And they are wonderful for an extra element when you are layering and mixing prints. If you have a beautiful print scarf it can give you inspiration for the colours that go together and how they can be colour blocked. It prompts you to elevate your outfit.

Always carefully unpick the label. Whether it's from Hermès or H&M, the label will always somehow make its way to the front.

Bags

I don't think I know a single woman who has fewer than five bags. I won't suggest even more to buy, as bags will suit different lifestyles and symbolise different things to different people. But the bags I think everyone will find useful are, a black bag, a metallic bag (see page 254), a neon bag and a cross-body bag.

Belts

These can help evolve any outfit (see page 268). The best belts are often vintage purchases, as you can find fantastic quality for a very good price.

Jewellery

It's never about how much things cost. I have inexpensive high street and designer pieces and I would no more part with either. Perhaps you are someone who will use one beautiful piece to bring an outfit together and elevate it. Or you prefer to go for subtle continuation of the tones, reflected in your earrings, your shoes, your bag. Or introduce a pop of contrast.

- When I'm looking at what earrings will look best on a woman, I look at the angles of her face and the length of neck. We have a space below our ear and our jawline. Think about how to fill that space.

- If you have a long, thin neck, try an architectural earring that fills in that space. It will frame your face and adds structure.

- If you have great cheekbones, celebrate them with a diamond shaped earring as it will add to that line. A teardrop shape will flatter most of us if it's in the right size.

- Big or delicate can depend on your character. If you are a glasses wearer you might find it hard to get around a potential clash with big earrings and people with very delicate features may not suit overwhelming items. Do experiment.

- Vintage jewellery allows you to find pieces that no one else has. The rule of thumb for me is that if the era of the jewellery and your age has more than forty years in difference, then it might be best to not wear it on bare skin. Over fabric, it will look very different and feel modern.

- I love layering necklaces. You can come up with all different combinations, and a more classic string of pearls can be made modern with the addition of a gold chain necklace.

- For bangles, mix up the widths to add texture and interest.

- If you have a necklace the wrong length, make it longer by putting two necklaces together clasp to clasp.

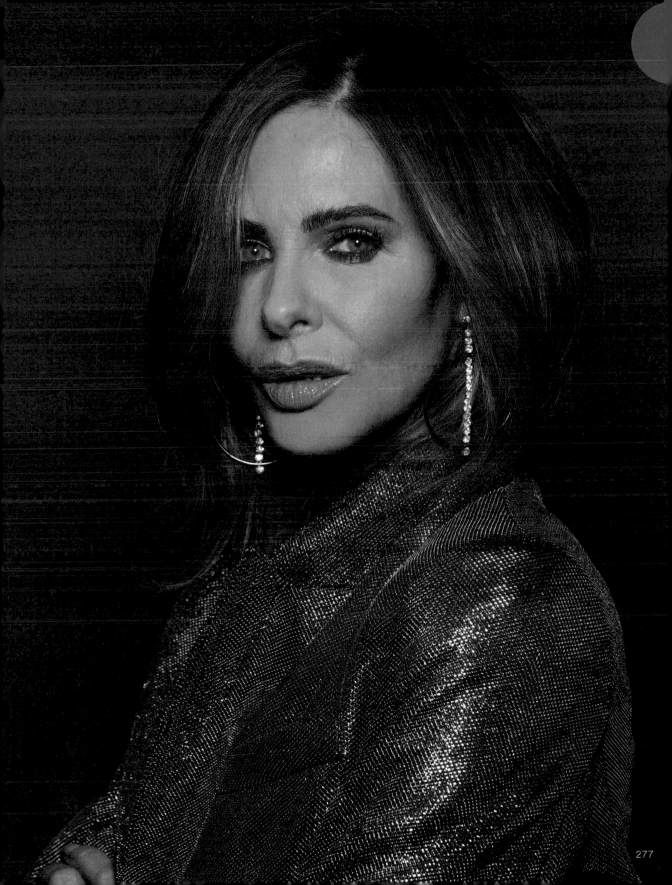

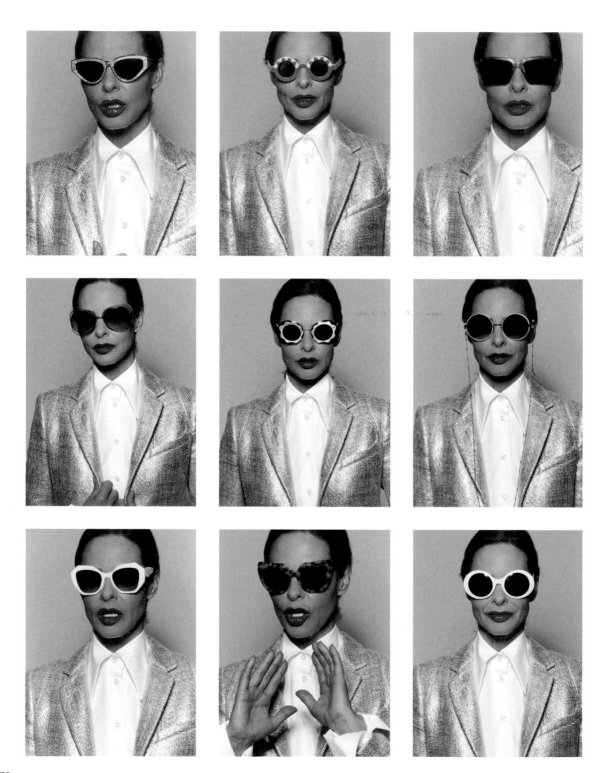

Sunglasses

This is where you can have some fun as they really can bring a hit of joy to your day (see page 260). You can definitely throw out some of the glasses rules (see page 206). A mad pair of sunglasses will change your whole look.

Lens quality

If want to buy a quality pair of sunglasses, look out for those that have a CE or UV400 mark on the frame. UV400 will protect your eyes from 99% of UVA and UVB rays. CE means that the lenses comply with EU safety standards, but do not offer as much protection as UV400. A polarized lens will reduce glare from surfaces that reflect light, which will help you see more comfortably when you're outside.

Storing your glasses

Do try not to throw your glasses in the bottom of your handbag where they will get scratched - we want to look after things that we love so they last. Invest in a fun case if this will encourage you to use it. If you have multiple pairs, store them where you can see them. There is nothing sadder than a fabulous pair of sunglasses languishing forgotten in the drawer. There are plenty of inexpensive storage solutions designed specifically.

Reading glasses

Those of you who wear glasses to read - join me over here for a moment. Everyone else, carry on. If you need reading glasses, for goodness' sake make them fun! We can age ourselves when we see our reading glasses as a boring necessity and not as a style opportunity. When I put on my chocolate velvet glasses with a leopard print arm in a meeting, I am making a statement and it gives me presence in the room. This is the perfect example of where you can raise your baseline. Don't settle for ugly or dull.

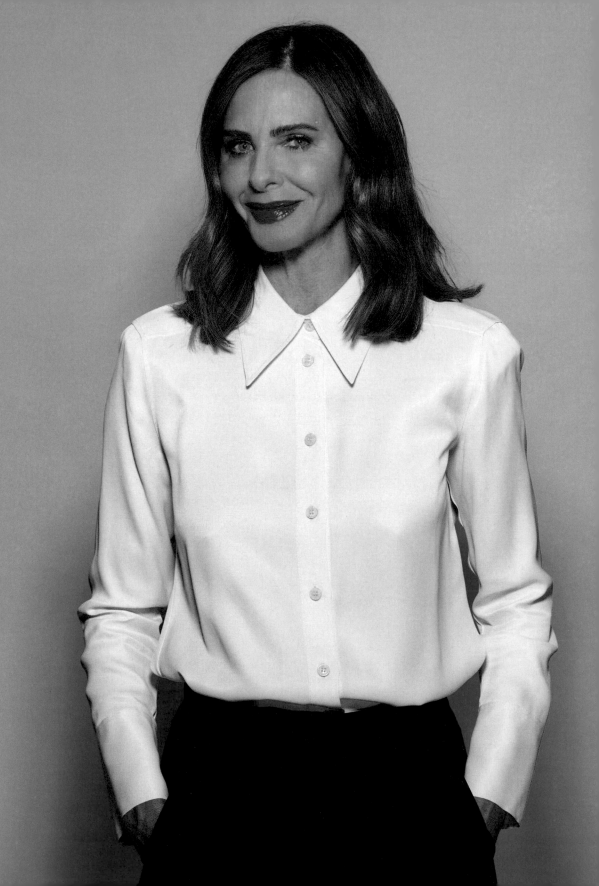

A basic white shirt styled eight ways

I hope that all of this talk of prints, colours and non-essential essentials has inspired you to look at your wardrobe in a brand new way. But how can we make the items we love work even harder for us?

Most of us have will have a white shirt (or cream or ecru - whatever is your shade) in our wardrobes and this is an item that gives us lots of options. So I challenge you to get out that faithful friend and see if you can find eight different ways to style it.

A note on collars

If you have delicate, small features, collars can be overwhelming for you. Something much simpler and cleaner is more likely to be your friend.

The simpler the shirt, the easier it is to style. If you gravitate to a more feminine style of dressing you might like to do a large collar done up but if you are more angular or you have big boobs this may feel a bit much for you.

A chic look that works for many women is wearing a shirt with a small collar over a high round-neck T-shirt, with just the top button done up. This gives you a sharpness around the face that will flatter many shapes.

Make the items we already own work even harder for us

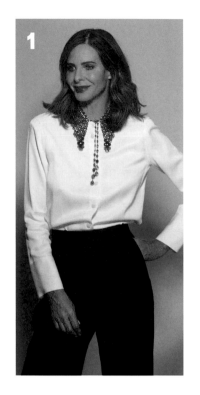

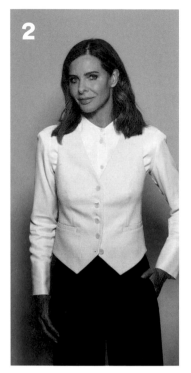

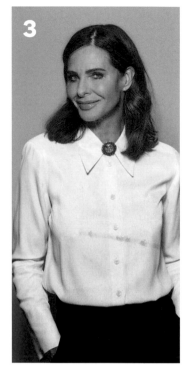

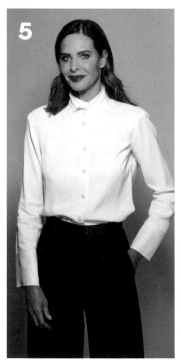

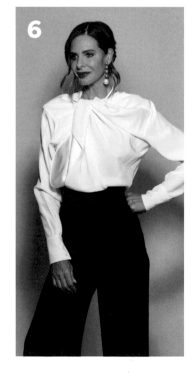

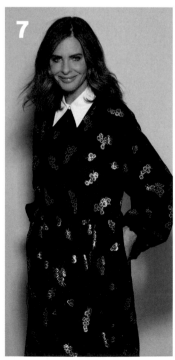

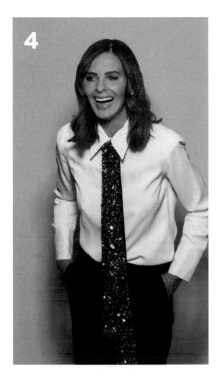

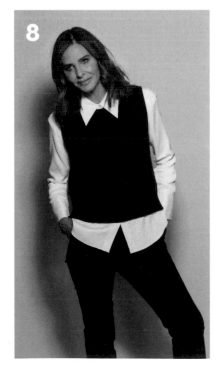

1 Collar necklace
Tucking in your collar and adding any necklace will turn this from day to night.

2 Waistcoat
Will enhance your shape and add structure.

3 Earring as a brooch
The perfect use for a single clip on earring.

4 Sequin scarf
A thin scarf as a tie creates a focal point.

5 Collar up
Stand your collar up and twist one edge underneath the other to create structure.

6 Twist
Face your shirt and twist it over at the neck. Put your arms in, with the shirt front to back. Fasten the buttons at the back.

7 Under a dress
This will dress down a too smart shirt.

8 Under a top
Wearing a top over will create a waistline.

Transform from night to day

How often do you look in your wardrobe and see the dresses and pieces that you have spent the most money on and yet worn the least?

You are going to feel so much better if you can find a way to dress them down and wear them more. They will become an investment, rather than an unjustifiable extravagance.

If something is truly fabulous then it deserves to be worn, so I want you to challenge yourself to do just that and make them a part of your everyday wardrobe.

On the following pages I have given a few ideas for how to dress down a more statement piece, but use the rules of layering (see page 272) and print (see page 238) to experiment further. This can be a really joyful process where you can develop your style and use a beautiful piece to work out what suits you.

Something fabulous deserves to be worn

Sequin dress

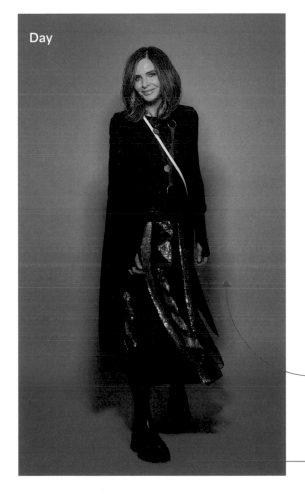

Day

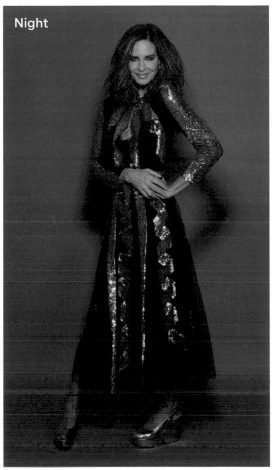

Night

Layering the dress is key. A gilet is good for this as it turns a dress into a skirt, and reduces the amount of sequin that is on show.

Pay attention to the shoe that you choose here. It should ground the dress and make it day wear. I have used a chunky black boot and dark tights.

Smart shirt dress

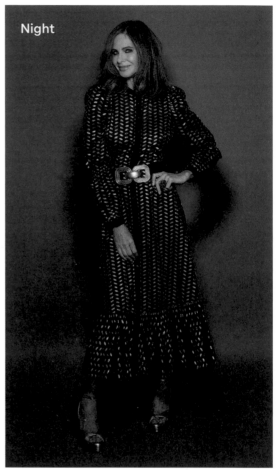

Night

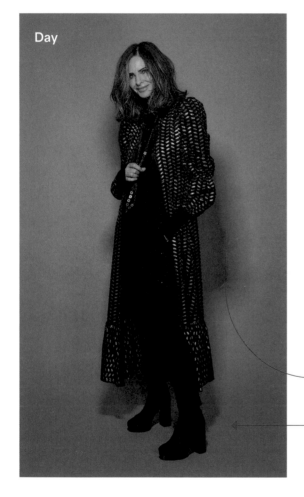

Day

Open those buttons!
Make it a coat-dress.

Think of the dress as a coat and
consider how you layer and style
your every day outfit underneath.
I have chosen a black outfit,
which the coat-dress then lifts.

Sequin jumpsuit

Day

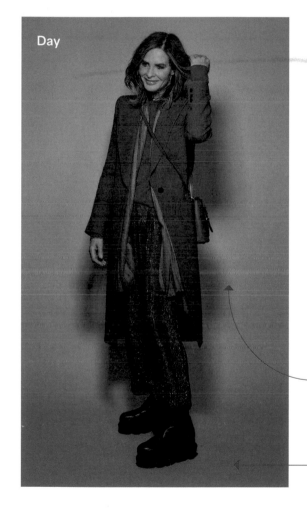

Night

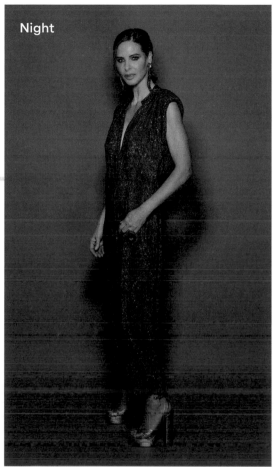

Wear a jumper underneath to quickly transform this piece. Alternatively, put a jumper on top, so that it turns them into a trouser.

Wear a trainer or a chunky boot, depending on the season. Add a draped scarf, a tailored coat and a cross-body bag to add layers and downplay the more standout item.

Bright silk dress

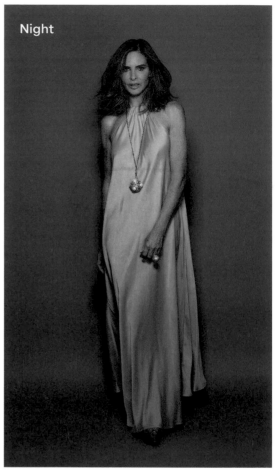

Night

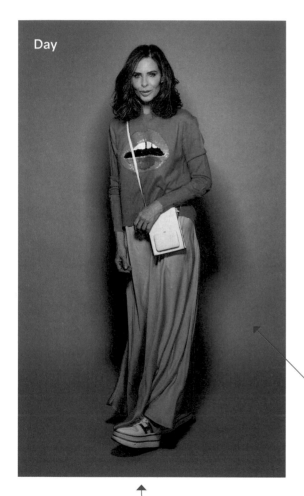

Day

What makes this work is choosing an equally bright colour for the jumper. Is should complement your dress. If it was in a strong or clashing colour, it would still be read as a dress.

Having an emblem on the jumper will help to play the look down and create a more relaxed feel. Wear with white trainers and a simple cross-body bag to bring a casualness to the silk.

Silver trousers

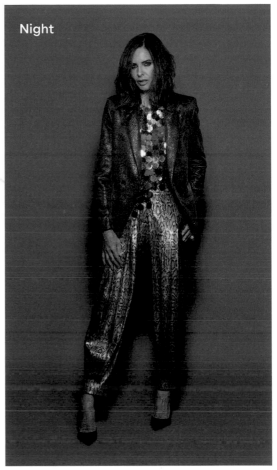

Night

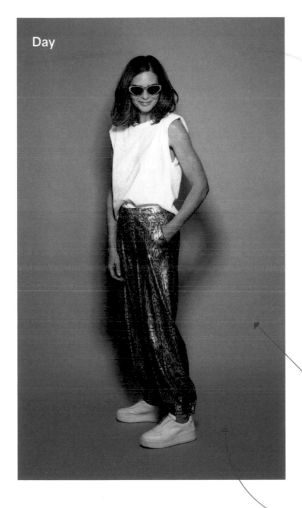

Day

I actually wear these more as a daytime look, and bought them with this intention. When you look at smart occasion items in a store, think instead about if they could be the hidden gems that will elevate any of your daytime pieces.

Always pair with more casual items such as a T-shirt, a sweatshirt and a white trainer to allow you to get away with it.

Embracing your style

I want you to dress with confidence and intention, to bring energy to your day and not be afraid to be seen. And to me, that means embracing every part of who we are in what we wear and how we wear it.

The women I have met and dressed over the years have shown me there are some core 'style personalities'. This is where our character, the clothes and accessories that bring us joy, and what we want to project into the world, come together.

There will be a style personality that most closely reflects how you like to dress, but you may find inspiration in a number. There may well be one or two where you think, 'that's not me at all'. But the reality is, we are all multi-faceted and the most confident of us will draw on elements of each. We feel different things more strongly on different days. This is about so much more than clothes. It's about the energy we project out into the world. My intention here is to do two things:

1   **How can you lean into your style personality and elevate your outfits further? How can you wake up your style?**

2   **I also want you to challenge yourself to look at other styles that don't necessarily reflect how you usually dress day to day and ask - what can I take from them and use?**

If you favour sharp tailoring, you probably don't have many floaty feminine dresses. But is there a part of you that would like to embrace an element of something softer and more relaxed? If you love Boho Chic then a Minimalist style may not immediately appeal, but it will give you the opportunity to introduce cleaner elements. And we can all benefit from recognising what makes us feel sexy and see how we can bring in touches of that, whatever our style or stage in life. This is about reawakening things you thought you'd lost and finding things you never thought you had.

The 7 style personalities

01 MINIMALIST

Understands shape and line to a tee; strips back any unnecessary detail.

02 MODERN CLASSIC

Drawn to great tailoring and clean lines but wakes it up with fresh cuts and accessories.

03 SOFTLY FEMININE

Loves pretty prints and soft romantic shapes.

04 ALWAYS SEXY

Body confident dresser who owns their sexuality.

05 ROCK CHIC

Daring and edgy, they channel the spirit of late nights and loud music.

06 BOHO

Embraces the cool, colourful and unusual in a laid back way.

07 ECLECTIC

Takes joy in combining prints, texture, colour and shape in unexpected ways. Unafraid to push the boat out and be noticed.

Layering not flow

Minimalism is all about layering. The lines and cut of each individual piece are important, but so too is how they work together. There might be a simple detail of a double cuff or texture in a sweater but nothing stands out; it's all about how the outfit works as a whole. It's a very structural, sleek look with a certain flow to it.

Minimalist makeup

The basis of Minimalist makeup is a clean face. A Minimalist might do a red lip but the focus is on detail and enhancing what is there, rather than adding lots of elements. So, of course, the base is important but so are the eyebrows. Add subtle highlighter to the high points of the face and use a neutral eye shade and carefully sculpted lashes to bring out the eyes, rather than too much colour.

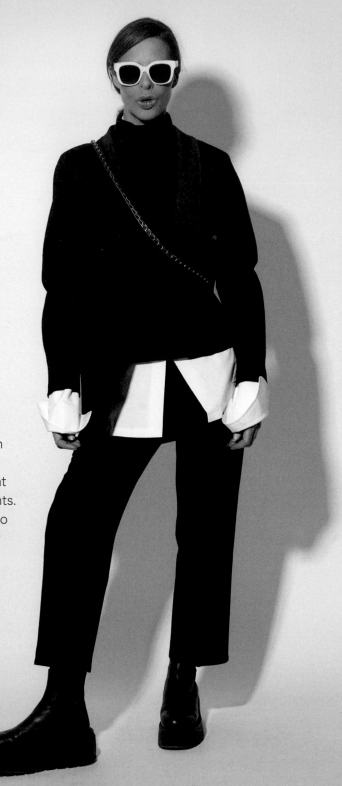

A few key pieces

A Minimalist wardrobe will generally be
compact and monochrome. I used: a
white shirt, a black trouser, a black jacket,
a T-shirt, a jumper, a gilet, brogues,
a chunky heel and a cross-body bag.
Everything is carefully chosen and
earns its place. I created 24 looks
with just 9 key pieces. More is
unnecessary as most things will
work together. A Minimalist will
wear jewellery but it will be classic
and pared back. It could be a silver
cuff or even the chain on a bag.
Hair should be sleek.

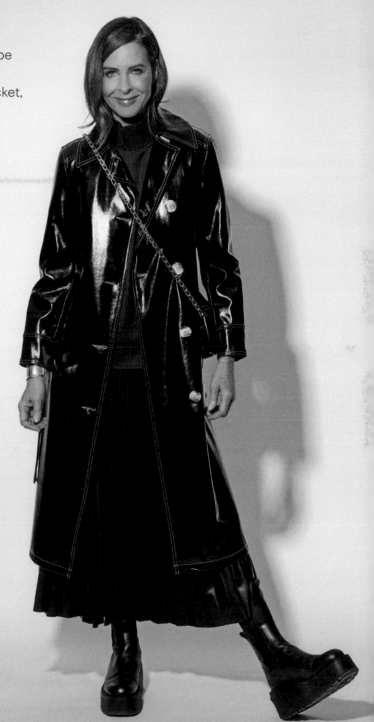

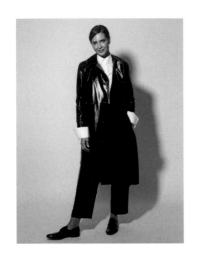
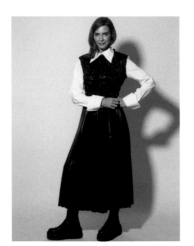
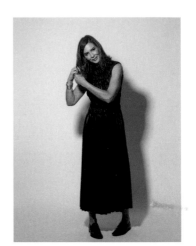
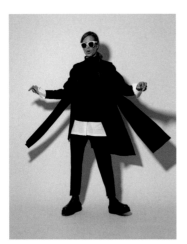
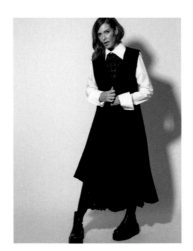
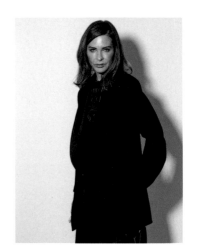
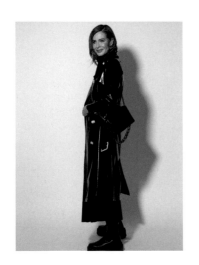
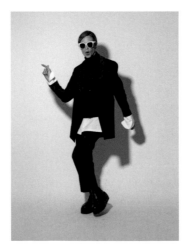
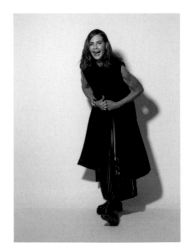

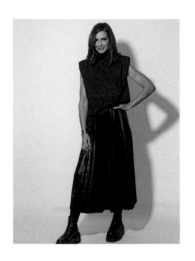
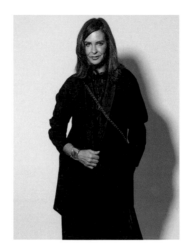
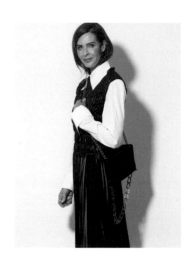
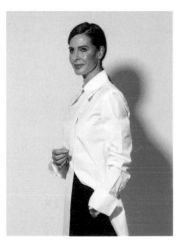
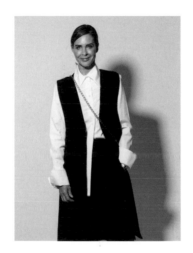
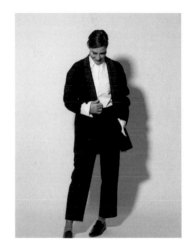
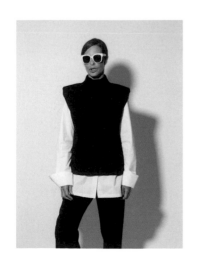
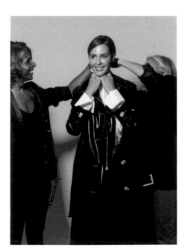
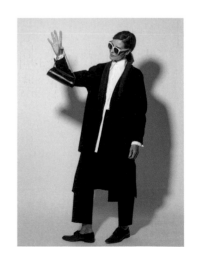

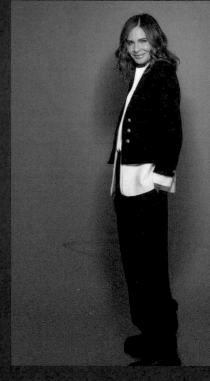

MODERN CLASSIC

If you are a Modern Classic then you appreciate what a well-cut jacket or trouser brings but know how to bring it alive with a couple of cool details. You probably don't have an overstuffed wardrobe and your clothes all look good together. You love good fabrics and are more likely to buy one really good suit than three that are just fine. You always look put together and may lean towards monochrome or a tonal palette. You always manage to look fresh and modern. You will tend to avoid prints. This is the epitome of ageless dressing.

You could do this if...

1   You save up for a few key, well tailored pieces.

2   You like to feel classic, but not dated.

3   You love a refined palette.

4   How you dress is all about structure and shape.

Find the joy

The structure of a Modern Classic wardrobe will give you great posture and allows you to present yourself with confidence. This style is much easier to wear as you only need a few key pieces, with tweaks made to the accessories rather than complete outfit overhauls. You will buy less and invest better, which is good for your wallet and the sake of the planet.

Accessorise

Use one or two accessories to direct
attention without letting them clutter
an outfit or steal the show. Coco Chanel
said, 'before you leave the house, look in
the mirror and take one thing off.' I tend
to disagree of course (personally, I put
something else on) but if you feel your
accessories are fighting each other or
there's too much going on, then you
can take a leaf out of the modern
classic style guide and focus on two.

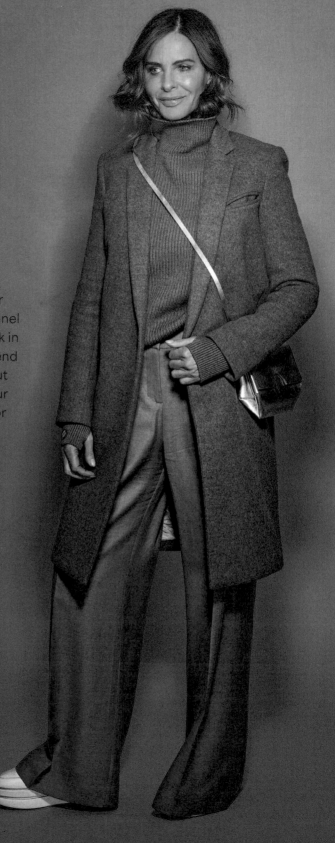

Appreciate
good tailoring

Whatever your style personality, having a
well-cut coat and jacket in your wardrobe
is always a necessity. That one piece can
pull jeans and a T-shirt together. It is about
a firm line across the shoulder and the
structure that the lapel brings.

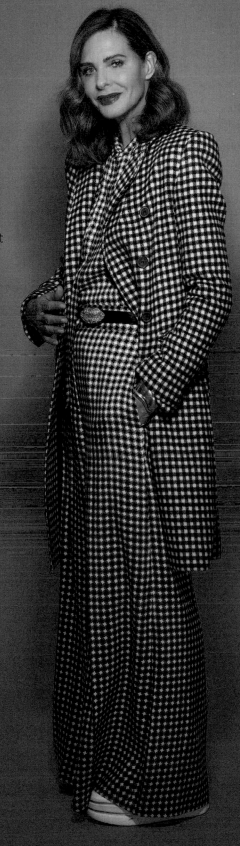

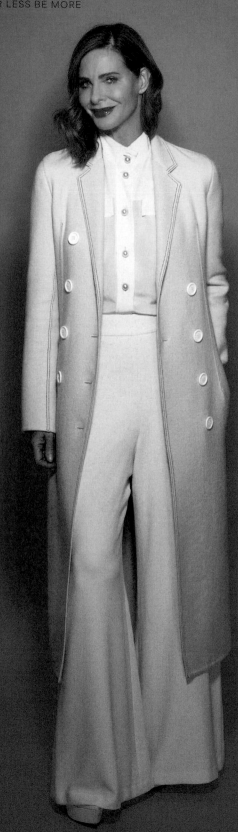

One colour dressing

There is nothing more chic than different textures in the same colour. Be sure to pick items with a good structure and cut, and consider how the items layer together to ensure a good flow.

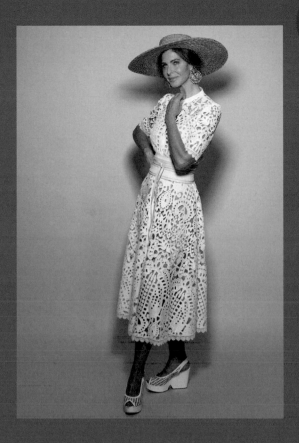

SOFTLY FEMININE

This style is defined by a beautiful delicacy. It's epitomised by small prints - think buds and sprigs rather than a whole flower - in soft shades. Chiffon, silk, lace and broderie anglaise are all staples for this look. The beautiful drape you get with some of these fabrics is particularly important, as being Softly Feminine means emphasising your waist. Just remember to use tonal colours to help an outfit flow.

You could do this if...

1	You love a small print.
2	You love soft and delicate fabrics.
3	You love the heroines in 1940's movies.
4	You are feminine, but not 'girly'.

Find the joy

If you have spent your life being a bit girly, this is the way to elevate and make your look that little bit more grown up. Conversely, if you have never been feminine in the way that you dress and are fearful that it will make you look too girly, this is a way to slightly soften your look without giving up the elements you already love.

Layer

The beautiful light fabrics that are key to this look are perfect for layering as they won't create bulk. The fabric should include small sprigs. If you are someone who prefers not to show their upper arms you can add another top under a split tulip sleeve. You can also wear trousers under a dress with slits up the side. Just remember that the colours will need to be tonally the same and be careful that nothing cuts you off across the ankle or swamps you around the waist.

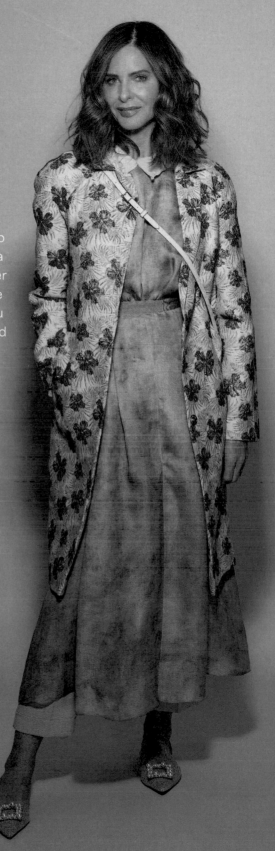

Lightness and lift

Appliqué and broderie anglais are this
styles best fabric friends. The colour
palette of softly feminine is oyster,
pastels, white, pale gold and silver. Take
this lightness up into the face by placing
highlighter under your base for an extra
glow. Wear blush higher up on the
cheekbones than you might usually
do. Pearls or other white earrings
will bring light next to your skin.

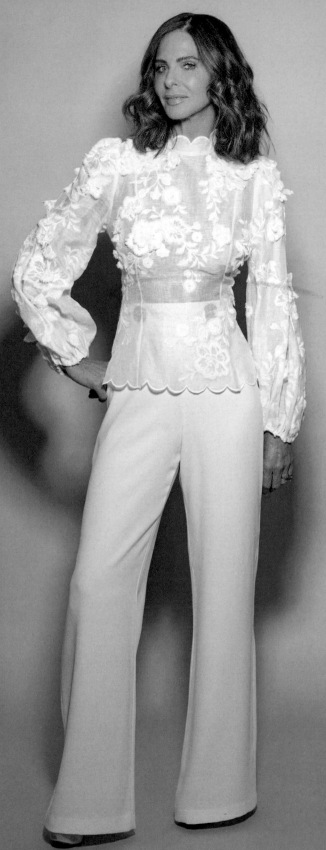

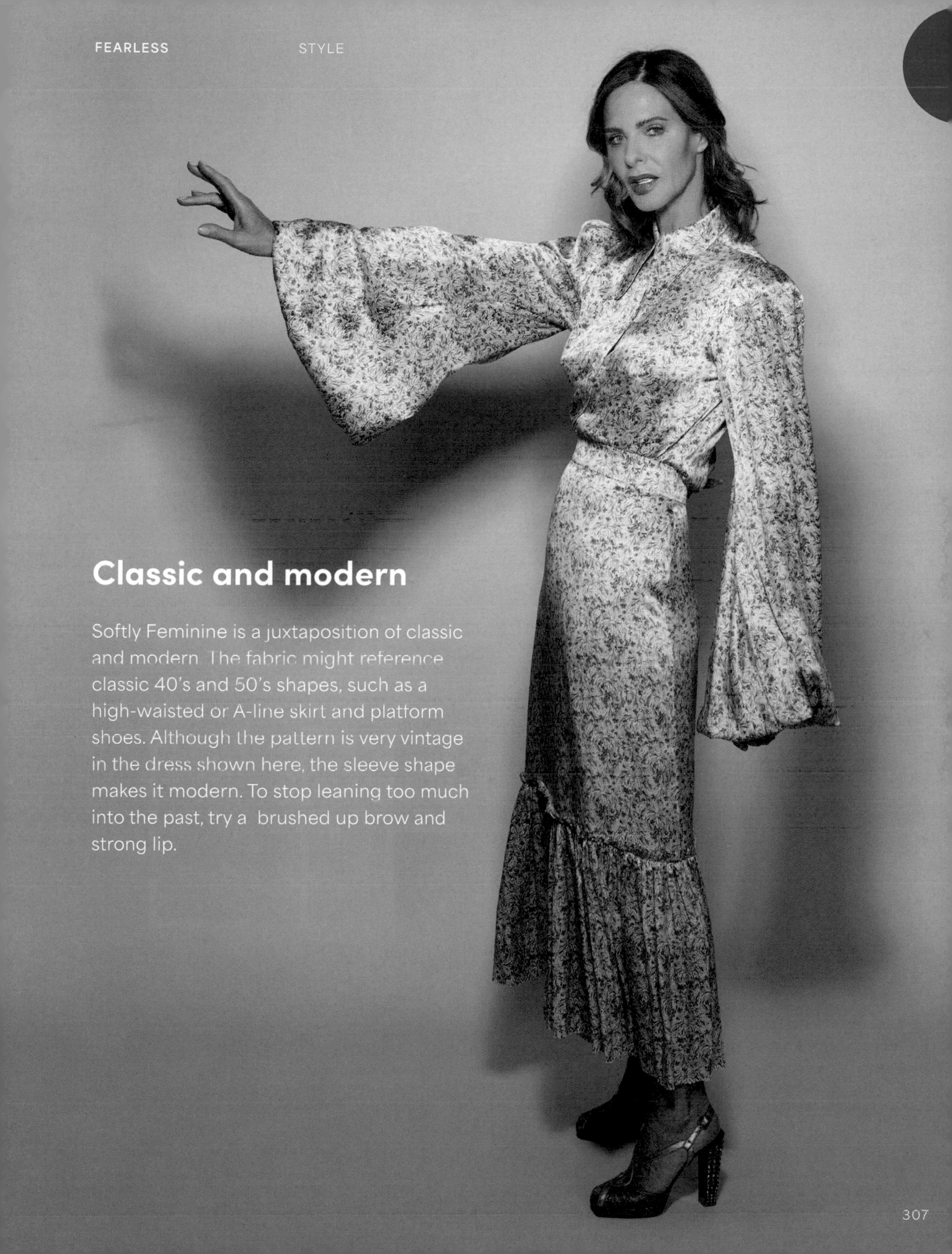

Classic and modern

Softly Feminine is a juxtaposition of classic and modern. The fabric might reference classic 40's and 50's shapes, such as a high-waisted or A-line skirt and platform shoes. Although the pattern is very vintage in the dress shown here, the sleeve shape makes it modern. To stop leaning too much into the past, try a brushed up brow and strong lip.

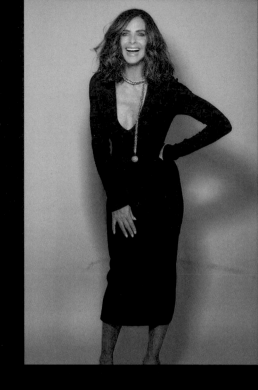

ALWAYS SEXY

'Sexy' in terms of what we wear means different things to different people. But what it comes down to is celebrating your body with clothes that are the perfect fit and directing the viewers' attention to exactly where you want it to go. Feeling sexy is about feeling in control. I believe it comes down to personality as to the extent to which you push this.

You could do this if...

1   You know what your assets are.

2   You are comfortable with a suggestive reveal.

3   You love skirts and trousers with a really good fit
and avoid excessive volume.

4   Your clothes can project what you might not
be confident enough to say.

Find the joy

I challenge every woman to try this look. This was the look I least
wanted to photograph, but it was actually the style I learnt the
most from. By pushing my boundaries, I opened myself up to the
idea that I could be sexy, which I never really thought I could be.
It really is crucial to try on different styles and see how you feel in
them. You might just surprise yourself.

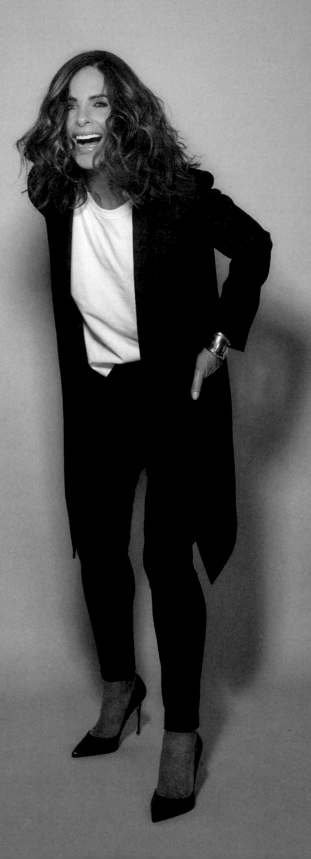

Sexy can come as a hint

From a distance, this feels like it could sit in Modern Classic, but the trousers are leather and the shoes are stiletto. This makes the look immediately sexy just from the connotation of the texture and shape of these versions.

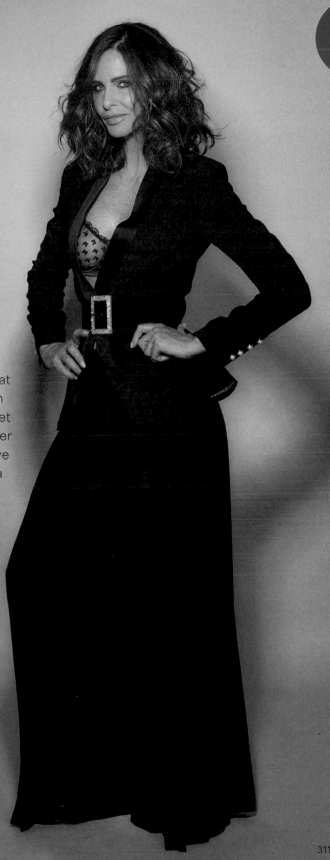

What's underneath

Sexy is all about hints and suggestions,
rather than everything being on show. That
could be a flash of a black bra underneath
a man's style white shirt or a tailored jacket
with just a bra on underneath, held together
with a belt to cinch in the waist. If you have
a proper cleavage, a deep set balcony bra
will lift the boobs and continue the fabric
to the waist to create an unbroken line.
But for those who are more flat chested,
the sheerness of a bra will feel sexy.

All in the eyes

Always Sexy has a mesmerising eye. If, like me, you have smaller eyes and a bigger face, it is worth taking the time to do an eyeliner flick or a softly smokey eye. Think about sheer metallics on the lid (with a dot of highlighter on the inside corner for added glamour) and black eyeliner along the waterline. Red lipstick can work for this look, but also consider a more mysterious brown or even a neutral, leaving all the drama to the eyes. Your hair should be undone but not neccessarily as messy as it would be in Rock Chic.

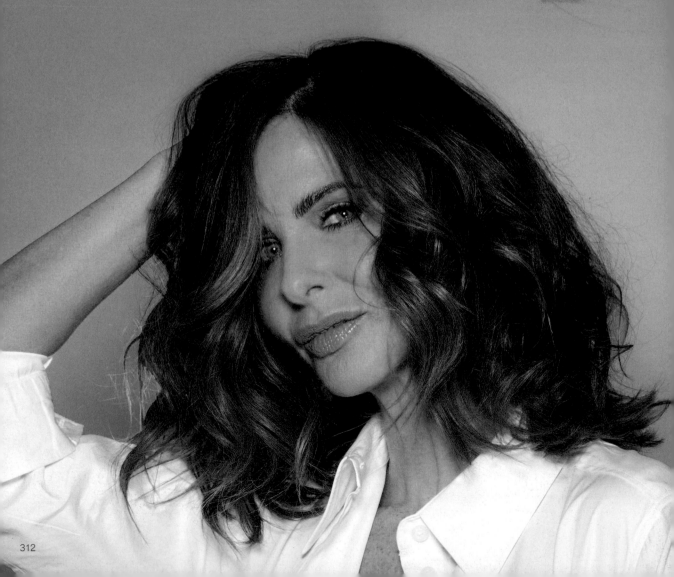

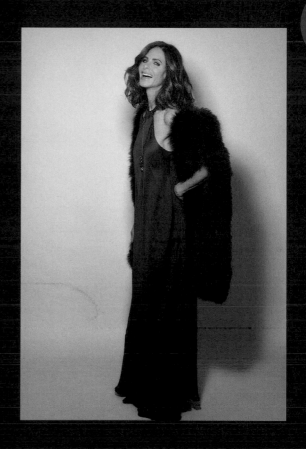

ROCK CHIC

Many women secretly desire to channel Rock Chic.
Eponymous, iconic women like Jane Birkin and Kate Moss
made this look popular, with their devil-may-care attitude.
If you are slightly down the path of life, you may feel that this
look is something that you can't do, but I have met women at
the age of 70 who channel this to perfection. It is naughtier
than any other personality and a very striking way of dressing.

You could do this if...

1   You want a new way to feel sexy.

2   You don't like to look like you have taken too long to get ready, but you still want to look good.

3   A black leather jacket is your favourite thing in the wardrobe.

4   You can't let go of your skinny jean and you need a new way to wear it.

Find the joy

You know you have got this look right when you feel very cool and very confident. And we all want that feeling in our life. There is something very appealing and achievable about this look, it really does feel fearless.

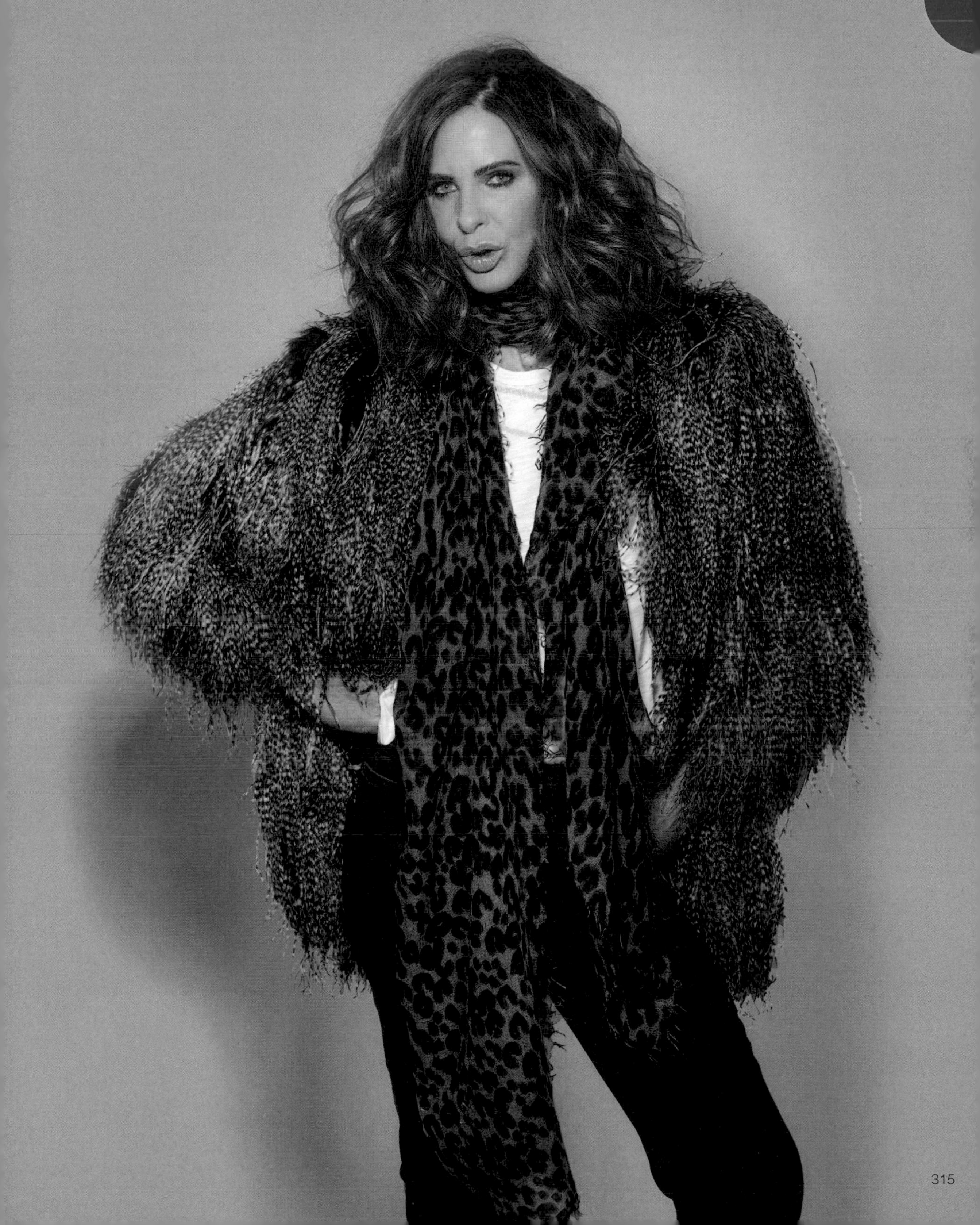

Soft tailoring

The Rock Chic takes inspiration from
the tailoring of the seventies, but the
difference is that the clean waistcoat
won't be embroidered and the shirt
underneath will be sheer and sexy
rather than a high frill.

Undone is better
than perfect

Rock Chics mainly come out at
night (although they still own fabulous
sunglasses) and they don't spend ages
getting ready. There will always be
something Rock Chic about a smokey
eye, a hint of shimmer and messy hair.
Think about your cheekbones and using
highlighter to emphasise them, though
Rock Chics aren't bothered about blush
– they don't want to look too healthy!

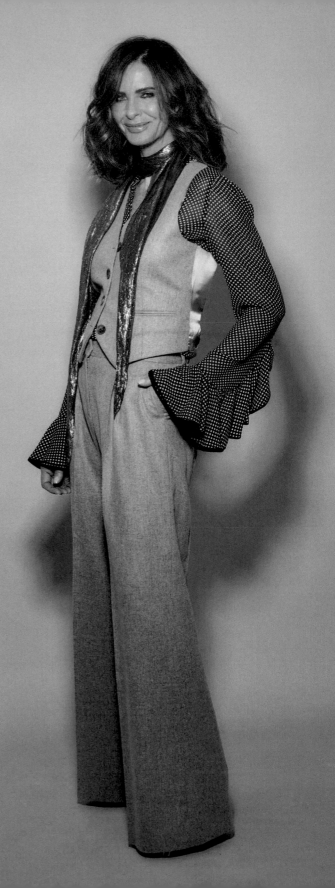

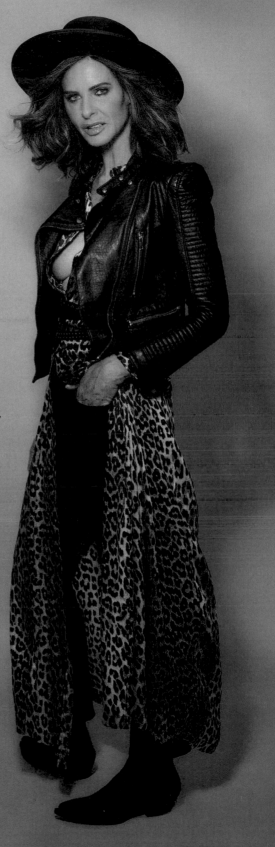

It's all about the jacket

Whether that's a boxy faux fur jacket,
a trench or the classic leather, a lot of the
cool factor of this style is embodied in the
right jacket. A good pair of boots helps too,
but a Rock Chic can just throw on a great
jacket over jeans and a T-shirt and be
good to go.

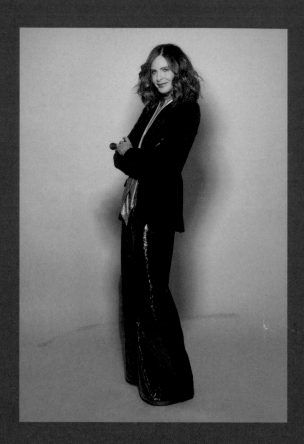

BOHO

You probably have a great eye for colour and print and you love the relaxed style and the opportunity for creativity that Boho brings. When we create a look from a specific era, we always want to make it live in the modern day. The Boho dresser can marshal vintage finds and modern pieces in different colours and patterns and turn them into effortless-seeming outfits.

You could do this if...

1   You can be quite whimsical.

2   You love to wear print.

3   You love the seventies.

4   You like to stand out from the crowd.

Find the joy

It is impossible to dress Boho and be uptight. You don't have to go with flowy items here, but the beauty of this style is that it will bring out your softer side. You can try out pattern clash and combinations that you have not tried before. I embrace this look when I want to feel slightly more feminine, as it is almost a safer way to feel slightly more sexy.

Print

The most important thing about wearing prints together is the silhoutte. Echo the shapes of the seventies. Embrace pattern clash. And be a magpie, drawing in different elements from different places. Boho women are good at unexpected combinations. Remember that you are looking for patterns that share two colours minimum and it's easier to mix prints that are of a similar size.

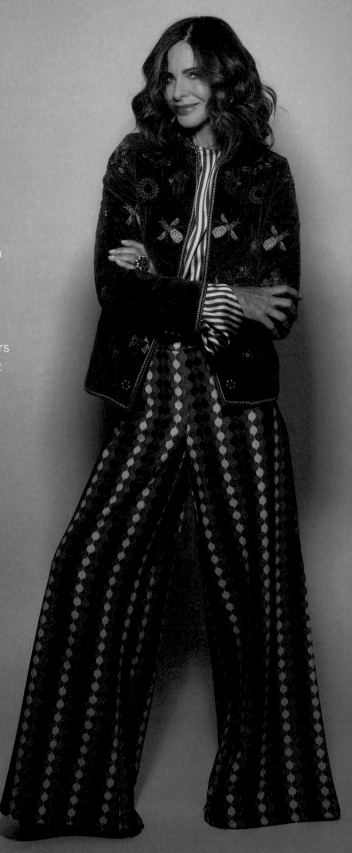

Flow

Boho is all about flow not structure. The long line of a trouser, the drape of a blouse, long layered necklaces, these all add a soft feminine touch. There's something deconstructed about it and never fussy. There's nothing uptight about Boho, so a glowing face and slightly messy hair is better than anything too 'done', you should look as if you have just got out of bed with the best hair. A bright red lip and the Boho style don't tend to suit each other.

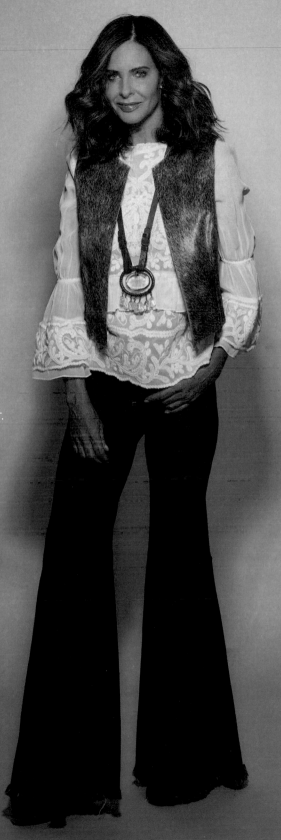

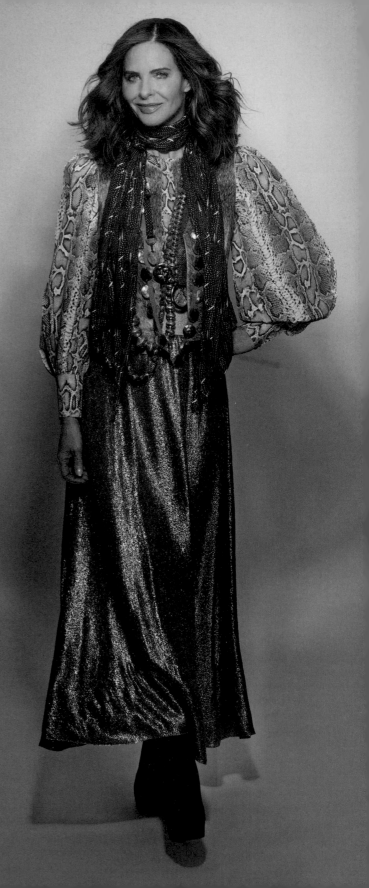

Glitz

It is a very joyful, rule-breaking approach to dressing. Embroidery, fringe, beading, applique ... all the details that would feel fussy to some of the other style personalities can be loudly celebrated here. Instead of a tailored coat, a faux fur or a velvet jacket – or even a cape – are good outerwear. Go glam in the winter with bright sequins and velvet.

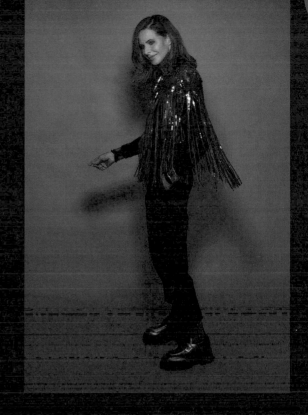

ECLECTIC

Eclectic style is the epitome of joyful, confident dressing. It's for people who love clothes, for whom getting dressed is never a chore and standing out is not a problem. It's about embracing texture in tweeds, faux fur and velvet; bringing in light with sequins, metallics and Lurex; and going for it with strong, eye-catching prints. There's definitely a luxe to this look – so cotton, soft jersey and Breton stripes have no place here. It is about having a healthy disregard for the rules. Eclectic women don't worry about conforming.

You could do this if...

1   You don't like to follow rules.

2   You express a different aspect of your personality in how you dress every single day.

3   You shop everywhere and will buy pieces entirely on their individual merit.

4   You would be described as a 'more is more' person.

Find the joy

For this look, you will need to let go of the rules of dressing and embrace the freedom to experiment. A great way to start dressing this way is to get out a clothes rail and display all of your most extreme items on it. There are no rules, just pull out anything statement that catches your eye. Now have fun and try to create a few different outfits using only these pieces.

Don't forget the face

Even in adventurous, creative dressing, there are still some fundamental principles at work. You don't want your outfit to wear you. This might mean upping the ante with your makeup – for example, bringing shimmer to your eyes and cheeks if you are wearing sequins or metallics – or being intentional about what you choose to wear right next to your face. If you are going luxe, think about your hair. A certain level of grooming is needed.

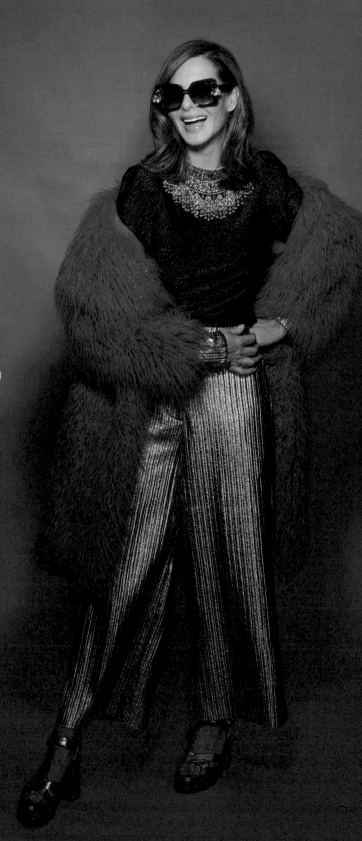

More is more, but ...

... it's about the right things in the right places. You want all the pieces to work together in one big happy choir, rather than fighting to drown each other out. You can absolutely layer, but think about all the details – right down to the gold sock or sequin cuff – rather than throwing it all on and hoping for the best. You still want to honour your shape and not get lost under all the fabulousness.

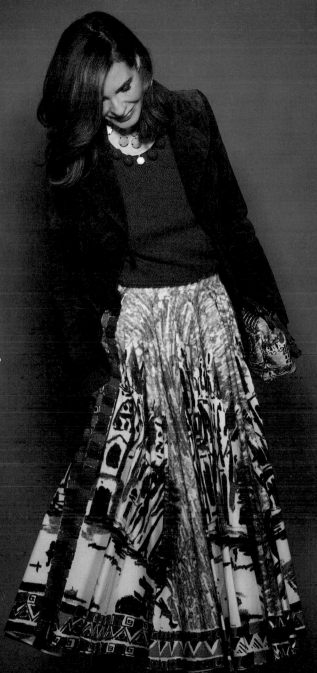

Don't rule anything out

Mix bright colours, textures and layer those prints. Everything can work everywhere, that is the joy of Eclectic. Don't worry too much about the specific occasion. Mix vintage, heritage and brand new pieces together to create a bold and exciting outfit.

How to organise

Now you know your style personality, it is time to look at how you organise. Arrange your wardrobe so that when you go to it you feel inspired. If it is dark and overstuffed then things will get lost and it will be harder to spark new ideas.

At the start of a season

Put away things you aren't going to wear. Use good storage boxes under the bed, under the stairs, on top of a cupboard ... Make sure everything is washed first and stored properly.

Arrange by colour and use

Consider separating pieces into rainbow colours, neutrals and prints. Then place workout gear and summer holiday clothes together, rather than clogging up the main wardrobe.

Hangers

Wire hangers are the enemy. They snag and get tangled when you're pulling things out in a rush. Consider using velvet effect 'huggable' hangers which are slim and don't take up space. Long, snap hangers are best for skirts as they don't have clips that get caught, while padded hangers are for anything soft or delicate.

Accessories

I am obsessed with small perspex boxes for storage. You will use your things more often if you can see them. With bags, whatever their cost, keep them stuffed so that they don't lose their shape (I generally use bubblewrap). I keep fabric bags wrapped up, so they don't become dusty and I stack hats on top of each other, crown on crown, so they keep their shape.

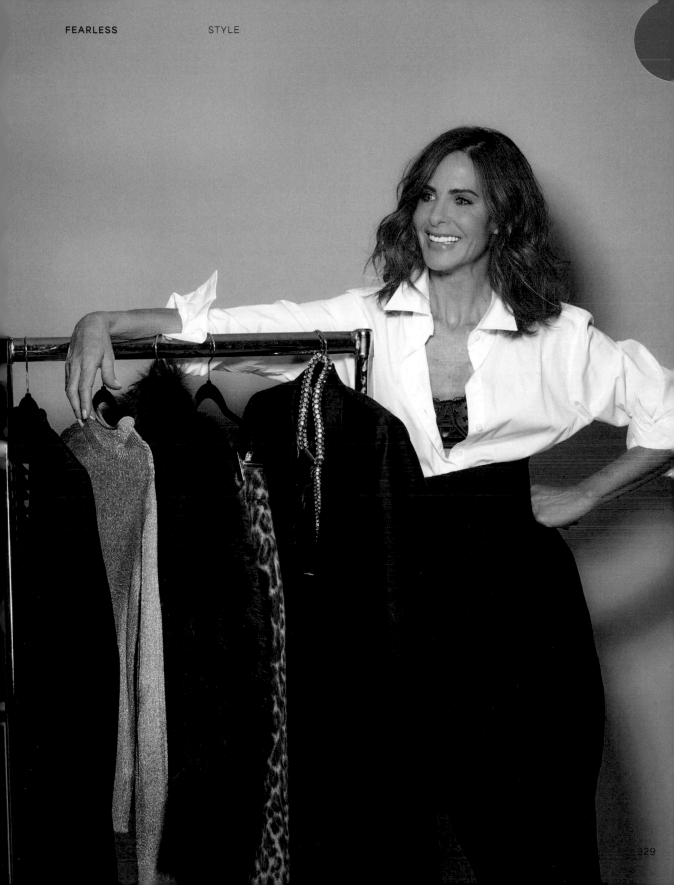

How to store your items

How I look after my things doesn't depend on what they cost me – it's about cherishability. I want to look at things I love, and make getting dressed a source of joy and not stress.

Jumper storage

These can be folded or rolled so they don't lose their shape. (If you hang one that is a touch short so it stretches, use a wide-armed hanger.) I handwash cashmere jumpers and lay them out on a towel, roll up and leave to mostly dry. When they are nearly dry, hang them over a banister or similar. I have inexpensive ones that have lasted years this way.

Moths

Moths are the absolute enemy. As you will well know if you have ever lost a cashmere jumper to their appetites. They have expensive taste and will only eat your most prized items. (Though it's actually the larvae that does the damage.) Putting items that are showing early signs of moth activity in the freezer does work but you will need to leave them there for up to five days to kill off the eggs too. Dry cleaning will also get rid of them.

Prevention is best. Keep the floor of your wardrobe hoovered as they love a dusty corner and invest in modern moth repellents. When storing precious clothes long-term, consider a zip lock bag.

Keep your white trainers white

You can put them in the washing machine on a short, cool wash with a low spin but it can be risky if it's not recommended by the manufacturer. I wipe Cif or Jif cream cleaner across the leather or plastic with a clean, damp sponge. Remove the product with a wet cloth and run them under the tap. Remember to wash the laces too, just place them in a delicate bag.

A note on underwear

There's no point in having beautifully cut clothes if you are wearing the wrong underwear underneath.

The knicker drawer

Get rid of uncomfortable, tatty knickers, they are not a good start to the day. Always have three seamless, simple pairs of knickers in your skin tone, as these will go under everything.

Bras

I could devote pages to bras and every woman will have a shape she feels most comfortable in. Years ago, Susannah and I did a bra show and 96 percent were not wearing the right one. Most will go one inch too big around the chest and one cup size too small. Our boobs do change shape as we go through life, so you may need to get refitted from time to time. If you have big boobs, wear a bra that lifts them up and separates, rather than flattening them or pushing them to the side. Remember the view will be different when looking at ourselves in the mirror. Don't feel you need to hide them, own those puppies!

Tights and socks

Ditch any saggy, bobbled tights and under no circumstances allow tights with a hole back into your drawer. Consider a range of sock lengths so that you can avoid any unappealing gaps between your trousers and your shoes. This creates an unbroken flow.

Slips

A nude slip can be very useful. Lots of dresses come with a cheap built-in slip, hardly ever in your skin tone, that cause static. Cut them out, wear a nude slip and it will look twice the price.

Making the cut

Before you begin a huge cull - which will be draining and may take a day - wash your hair and put on some makeup. You are going to be making decisions about what works and doesn't work for the woman you are so it's important that you feel and look good. You want to notice the contrast when you put on things that aren't right for you any more. And to see the good more clearly.

I highly recommend buying or borrowing a free-standing rail so you can hang things outside your wardrobe, where you can properly see them. Get everything out from the cupboard, the drawers, under the bed. All of it. And lay it out as much as you can. Do this in the living room if it's bigger and/or the light is better.

Goodbye pile

1   First deal with what doesn't fit. We need to dress for the body we have today and not the body we wish to have in the future. If you are constantly seeing clothes that are no longer your size, they will bring up memories and create a bad mindset. We all fluctuate in size. If you must keep some larger or smaller items, find a box and put them away somewhere.

2   Now you know what colours and tones you suit (see page 14), remove the extreme opposites of those colours. As you won't want to wear anything that isn't your best colour near your face, get rid of any top that is not your colour.

3   Turn to those things you do wear every day and look at them critically. If it's lost its shape or is faded or damaged in a way that's not fixable, it will make you feel tired when you put it on. If it's been a loyal favourite, make a note to replace it with something similar.

4 We all have sweatpants that we wear when we are feeling under the weather or on our period, and the jumper that reminds us of an old boyfriend. Just think about how you feel when you wear them. Is it time to move on and raise your baseline?

Keep pile

1 On your rail, hang the things that you do wear, are in good shape and work for the woman you are today.

2 Look at all the things you rarely wear but you don't want to get rid of. These are often the items that you bought for an event and cost you the most. You put them away because they are special, with the result that you've hidden them from yourself and you never see them as anything other than 'the dress for the wedding'. If you can't think of three ways to wear it, you should get rid. Challenge yourself to think how you can wear the item any day (see page 284).

3 You will have items that aren't quite right but you are reluctant to part with. Perhaps the fabric is fabulous but the length is unflattering. If the colour suits you, the quality is good and the shape generally works, these are candidates for a revamp (see page 334).

4 Finally, if you want to hold onto something for a daughter, or someone else, then find another place to safely store it away rather in your wardrobe, where it will get in the way.

How to revamp old friends in need of a lift...

When you did the cull, did you find things that you still love but that have an issue? This is where we give some love to our loyal old friends, reinventing them so they can continue to bring us joy.

For simple alterations, a local drycleaner will often do. For anything more complicated you will need to find a dressmaker/tailor who not only has the expertise but can advise you on whether the change will work the way you want it to. Here, I have given some old friends a new lease of life.

Show some love to your loyal old friends

A corporate suit

1 Fold the bottom of your trouser into your sock and tuck into a more modern boot to create a more flattering drape.

2 Add more shape to the outfit by adding a belt and tucking in your top.

3 Introduce statement jewellery or cuffs to draw the eye.

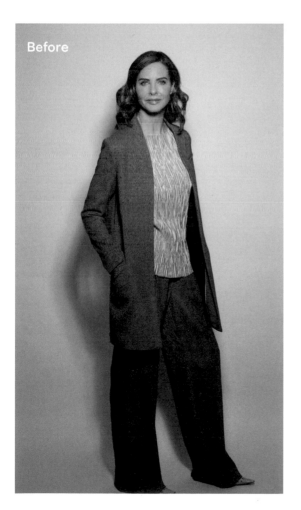

Before

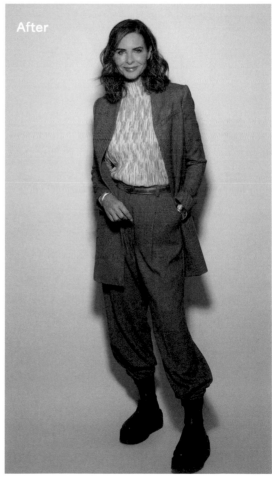

After

A dress in the wrong length

1 If the dress is too short, trim off any excess to create a fitted top that can be tucked into any trouser or skirt.

2 If the dress is too long, work out where the best length is on your leg and cut to sit.

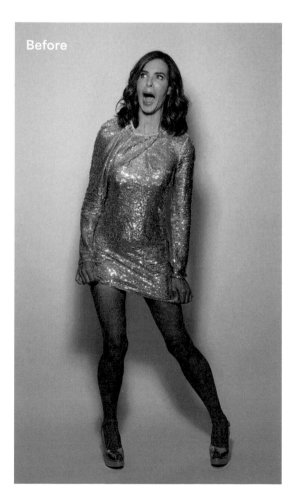

Before

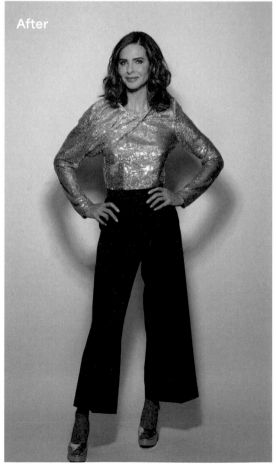

After

An ill-fitting coat

1 If the sleeves of your coat are too long or too short, one of the best ways to give it a new lease of life is to cut off the sleeves to create a gilet.

2 Be sure to leave in any shoulder pads. This will give the gilet a great shape.

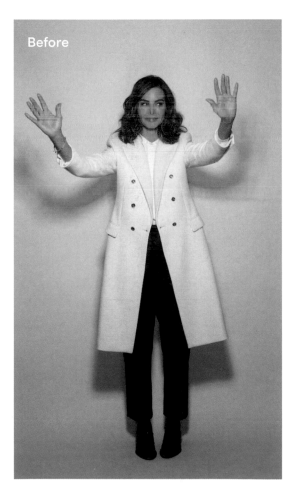

Before

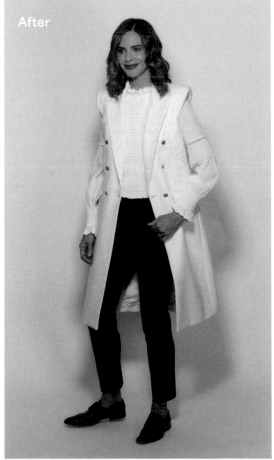

After

ASK YOURSELF

1 Is it the right shape but the wrong colour?

2 Is it the right colour but the wrong shape?
(unless it's a candidate for a revamp, see page 334)

3 Is it a fabric that you find irritating or it makes you sweat?

4 Is it too flouncy/frilly/busy for what you are channelling?

5 Does the sleeve make your arms look too long or short?

6 Does the print wear you, and you don't wear the print?
(see page 238)

7 Is it a holiday purchase that seemed like a great idea at the time but you're never going to wear?

8 Does it fit?

9 Will you never feel comfortable in it - is it itchy or are you always yanking down the hem?

CHALLENGE YOURSELF

1   Swap

Twice a year in the Trinny London office we have a party where we all bring in clothes we have fallen out of love with and swap them with each other. We play games to decide who gets to choose first. Consider cutting the labels off so you can't judge an item by cost, only on the merit of the item and if you love it. It's fun and a great way of finding new homes for items. You could organise a charity event or just get together with friends.

2   Donate

As well as traditional charity shops, there are organisations that take formal wear for girls going to school prom who may not be able to afford a dress, suits for women attending job interviews, coats for the homeless and many other things besides.

3   Sell

There are increasingly more ways to sell clothes online, whether they are designer, high street or preloved. Your love affair with an item might be finishing but it might be just what someone else is looking for and it is a simple way to make a little extra money from the clothes that you no longer wear.

How to shop without making mistakes

Now you know what colours, shapes and styles fit your personality, you can shop fearlessly. Wherever you shop, the principles are the same. Go with a focus and a purpose and be mindful of slipping back into old habits that don't serve you any more.

How you approach shopping depends on your personality. If you found a lot of never-worn clothes in the back of your wardrobe, it is likely you need to be aware of emotional grazing. Below are a few tips to help you.

Know your purpose

Starting off with one mission and ending with another is where we can often make mistakes. If you are out shopping for a dress for an event, focus on this task and don't get distracted by anything else. But if you are out shopping for fun with a friend, it might be time to experiment with new ideas and get someone else's help and feedback. Keep a list on your phone of the things you need to buy and the colours you suit.

Avoid emergency shopping

This is where we make the most mistakes. Charging around in a panic trying to find a dress to wear that evening is too much pressure to guarantee success. Weigh up how often you need a smart outfit, take a look at what you have in your wardrobe and make the purpose of your next shopping trip to buy those great going out outfits. Give yourself the time to fall in love with the dresses, give yourself options and you will always wear them with confidence.

Shopping online

I am absolutely guilty of occasionally doing a midnight online shop up when I can't sleep and sending back 90 per cent of it. We all fall into that trap, but it's rarely a good use of your time.

Treat online shopping like you would an appointment. Choose a time, mark it in your diary and sit down and do it intentionally, not distracted in the back of a cab. Emotional, rushed online shopping to give you a hit is just a bit too much like drunk texting - unlikely to end well.

How to shop

Every website will have a filter system. Before you scroll, decide what you are looking for and filter by size, print, colour. This will stop you getting distracted. Always only search for the size you are.

Sizing

Yes, it is sometimes hard to know what size to go for when we are shopping online, particularly with an unfamiliar brand. But increasingly, websites contain this information if you look for it. Know your own measurements - they are just numbers, it's no big deal and it can really help you to buy clothes that work for you without having to bother to return masses of stuff unnecessarily. Of course, sometimes the only information is 'the model is 5'10" and wearing a size 8', which tells you little other than she is very slim to have those proportions. If that is all you have to work with, consider how does it looks on her and gauge from that.

As a rule of thumb, designer fashion comes up smaller than the high street, with the exception of high street teenage brands, which will size up smaller than designer. Be aware that different ranges from the same brand will use different models for their sizing. If you have something already from a particular range, it might not be the same as something in a different range.

In store shopping

If you're ready for some targeted shopping to fill in those gaps you've identified in your wardrobe, here is my quick guide to tackling the high street:

Know where you're going

Make a beeline for four or five shops that work for your body shape and your budget. If you have time you can always try a few others.

Be prepared

Yes, the lighting in changing rooms is usually ghastly. There's not much you can do about this but you can go with makeup on, good hair, feeling like your best you. Take heels and bring shapewear.

Put your blinkers on!

Ignore anything that isn't your colour, shape, or fabric. Do try on before you buy to minimise having to sort out returns.

Take a picture

How we see ourselves in the mirror is often very different to how we see ourselves in a photo. We can be more objective.

Don't buy it there and then

It really helps if you sleep on it. It will allow you to realise how much you need it and want it.

Feel the fabric

Scrunch the fabric to see if it will crease badly. Is it static? Never compromise! If something isn't right, keep moving.

Shopping preloved

There are many wonderful reasons to hunt down preloved items online or in real life. First, of course, there's the sustainability aspect. We are all aware of the damage fast fashion is doing to the planet. It is yet another reason to value the things we already own, make them work hard and look after to them to ensure they remain wearable for as long as possible. Then there is the thrill of finding something unusual no one else has, of getting a bargain and the opportunity to buy a designer piece a couple of seasons old that was too pricy at the time.

There are more and more preloved sites cropping up all the time and where you head depends on what you are looking for. For example, Lyla has a talent for finding things she loves on Depop, whereas I can lose hours trawling Vestiaire Collective. Whatever you are drawn to, always bear in mind:

Condition

You don't want to allow something into your wardrobe that is already tired or starting to lose its shape. If you are shopping online and can't be sure then best to avoid.

Size

Get exact measurements from the seller. Sizes vary - particularly in preloved clothing.

Look after your items so that they remain wearable

Index

A little more advice

If you are looking for more help, do please reach out. Below are just a few resources that you might find helpful:

Mental health:

Anxiety UK
anxietyuk.org.uk

Mental Health Foundation
mentalhealth.org.uk

Mind
mind.org.uk

Samaritans
samaritans.org

Mental Health America
mhanational.org

National Institute of Mental Health
nimh.nih.gov

Mental Health Research Canada
mhrc.ca

Canadian Mental Health Association
cmha.ca

Addiction:

Alcoholics Anonymous
alcoholics-anonymous.org.uk | aa.org

Narcotics Anonymous
ukna.org | na.org

National Gambling Helpline
begambleaware.org

Shatterproof
shatterproof.org

Families for Addiction Recovery
farcanada.org

Relationships

Family Lives
familylives.org.uk

Relate
relate.org.uk

Lifestyle and beauty

Trinny London
trinnylondon.com/uk

Victoria Health
victoriahealth.com

The Tweakments Guide
thetweakmentsguide.com

Thank you to

Lisa Milton, Executive Publisher at HQ, who pitched me the idea of doing a book. Even though I thought I just wouldn't have the time, she made it easy for me to be able to do it.

My editor, Louise, who has the patience of a saint, and never loses her passion for perfection.

My dearest Michael, how we managed to survive each other for the last 25 years is a testament to how through thick and thin, you always have my back.

My rock, Weasie, I don't know where I'd be without you. You are the breakwater so that I can swim in a calmer sea. Molly, my Duracell bunny, who never stops unless a little accident defeats her and even then she can't stop moving; she is ever Joyful and a yes person.

Annie, I have done more shoots with you than I have shopped in Zara ... You are always patient, and you always make everything work. It is such a pleasure to work with somebody so in tune with one's own thought process that it becomes half the work and effort. Thank you to lovely Martha for always finding solutions during our manic book shoot too.

Dan, thank you for your glorious pictures and making me feel a little bit more ageless.

John, who can make whichever face I present to him my best face, and he always knows when I'm in need of a mood lift!

Greg, hair maestro, who is the foundation of my hair, and always sets me up for the day.

Kasun, our on set hair magician.

Ksenia, our lead engineer at Trinny London for helping
to figure out how to reverse our Match2Me algorithm and
make it work for the book.

Claire, our Chief Innovation Officer at Trinny London, who
inspires and educates me on skincare philosophy every day.

Kellieann, who was only meant to be helping on the
makeup section but stayed up late at night to work with
me on colour too.

To Liz, Lucy and Jess, for all their brilliant help with the
initial research.

Dr Erika, who has women's longevity at the forefront of all
the work that she does as a hormonal specialist. You taught
me how to live through hormonal change and to come out
feeling even stronger.

Victoria and Nathalie, who kept many of us going through
lockdown to be healthy with our bodies, and who have given
us wonderful tips for the book.

My dearest Shabir and Gill, the founders of Victoria Health, who
I have learned so much from in how we supplement and look
after our bodies. Your generosity in sharing your message so
that more people can get advice and direction is truly inspiring.

Jo and Sanjai, the two spiritual giants, who have taken us on
journeys of meditation.

Odete, who looked after me for quite a few years, and who was
the mummy when I needed one.

The whole team at HQ for their passion and vision.

Imagist for their gorgeous design.

The whole team at Trinny London, new and old, who work hard
every day so that women can always feel their best self.

And finally, the Trinny Tribe, a set of women who support and encourage one another to feel their best and who inspired me to write this book. You kept asking me to put all my advice in one place so here it is ... A huge thank you to all of you for sending us your glorious photos, I am sorry we couldn't use them all!

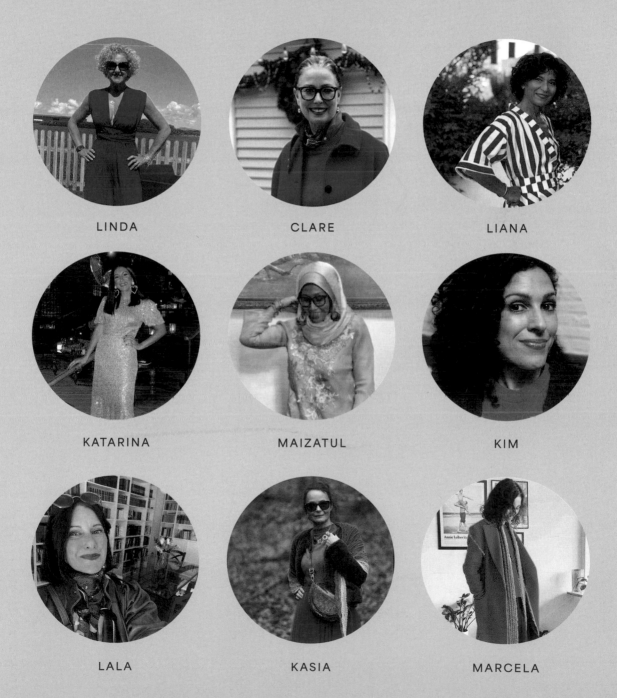

LINDA

CLARE

LIANA

KATARINA

MAIZATUL

KIM

LALA

KASIA

MARCELA

HQ
An imprint of HarperCollinsPublishers Ltd
1 London Bridge Street
London SE1 9GF

www.harpercollins.co.uk

HarperCollinsPublishers
Macken House, 39/40 Mayor Street Upper
Dublin 1, D01 C9W8 Ireland

10 9 8 7 6 5 4 3 2 1

First published in Great Britain by
HQ, an imprint of HarperCollinsPublishers Ltd 2023

This book is produced from independently
certified FSC™ paper to ensure responsible
forest management.

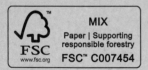

For more information visit:
www.harpercollins.co.uk/green

Printed and bound in Italy by Rotolito

Publishing Director **Louise McKeever**
Art Direction **Laura Russell**
Production Controller **Halema Begum**
Design **Imagist**
Editor **Liz Marvin**
Photography **Daniel Kennedy**
Stylist **Annie Swain**
Makeup **John Corcoran**
Hair **Kasun Godallawathga**
Researchers **Jess Beech** and **Lucy Carter**

All photography by **Daniel Kennedy** with the exception
of the images on pages 158, 213, 215, 217, 219, 221, 223,
225, 227, 229, 231, 233, 235, 237, 239, 240, 246, 249,
253, 256, 259, 263, 267, 271, 351, with thanks to the
Trinny Tribe.
And pages 20, 21, 22, 23, 24, 25, 40, 41, 42, 43, 44, 45,
with thanks to Trinny London Limited.